Therapeutic Exercises Using Resistive Bands

Caroline Corning Creager, P.T.

EXECUTIVE PHYSICAL THERAPY, INC.

BERTHOUD, COLORADO

Library of Congress Card Catalog Number: 98-093671
Creager, Caroline Corning

Therapeutic Exercises Using Resistive Bands.
Creager, Caroline Corning — 1st edition

Executive Physical Therapy, Inc.
P.O. Box 1319
Berthoud, CO 80513
(970) 532-2533
1-800-530-6878
e-mail: Caroline_Creager@unforgettable.com
website: www.CarolineCreager.com

Printed in the United States of America
1st Edition, 3rd Printing

The author has made every effort to assure that the information in this book is
accurate and current at the time of printing. The publisher and author take no
responsibility for the use of the material in this book and cannot be held
responsible for any typographical or other errors found. Please consult your
physician before initiating this exercise program. The information in this book
is not intended to replace medical advice.

ISBN: 0-9641153-4-4
Library of Congress Card Catalog Number: 98-093671

Book Design by Caroline Corning Creager

Composition by Alan Bernhard

Cover Design by Paulette Livers Lambert

Edited by Caryl Riedel

Drawings by Amy Belg

About the Author

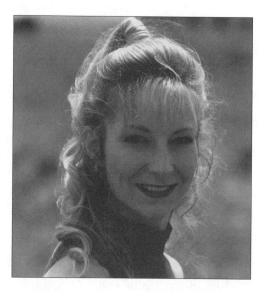

CAROLINE CORNING CREAGER, P.T.

CAROLINE CORNING CREAGER is an award-winning author and a nationally recognized lecturer on resistive bands, Swiss balls, and foam rollers. Caroline received her degree in Physical Therapy from the University of Montana in 1989. She is the owner of Executive Physical Therapy, Inc., in Berthoud, Colorado, and is a member of the American Physical Therapy Association, the Rocky Mountain Book Publishers Association, and the Colorado Independent Publishers Association. Caroline is the author of *Therapeutic Exercises Using the Swiss Ball, Therapeutic Exercises Using Foam Rollers, The Airobic Ball Strengthening Workout* and *The Airobic Ball Stretching Workout.* Her goal is to enhance health care professionals' understanding of how resistive bands can be used to facilitate individualized clinical, home, and work exercise programs.

Dedication

To my husband, Robert, for taking the time to model
for the front cover and *all* of the exercises in this book.
For his inquisitive nature to ask WHY? are you doing
the exercise this way, WHAT? muscles are firing
with this exercise, or WHEN? Are we going
to be finished taking photos.

To our newborn son, Christopher Robert Creager,
for sharing his charming smile, twinkling eyes,
and active vocal chords.

To my staff at Berthoud Living Center:
Kristi Blount, Haydee Contreras, Julie Herbert,
Valerie Kline, Nancy Meesey, and Donna Merritt,
for taking the time to make me laugh
during the endless days of bed rest
I endured for pre-term labor.

Acknowledgments

To Barbara Headley, M.S., P.T.,
for writing and sharing her knowledge
and expertise of electromyography
in the Electromyography Case Study One.

To Nancy Meesey, P.T.,
for contributing to the
Supine Exercises chapter.

To Leslie Vail, P.T.,
for writing and providing practical experience
to Case Study Two,
and for her persistence in asking me,
"When are you going to write and
publish a resistive band book?"

In Memory Of

MARY ELLEN GOLDBERG

and

ZORRI

My lovable dalmation,
running partner,
and
furry friend.
May she run in heaven
as she did here on earth.

Preface

After the success of my first two books in the Therapeutic Exercises Series, *Therapeutic Exercises Using the Swiss Ball*, and *Therapeutic Exercises Using Foam Rollers*, many clinicians approached me expressing an interest in a resistive band book similar in format to my other books. I subsequently took on the challenge and wrote, *Therapeutic Exercises Using Resistive Bands*.

The focus of *Therapeutic Exercises Using Resistive Bands*, is to improve individualized clinical, work, recreational, and home exercise programs by presenting illustrated and easy-to-read exercise instructions using resistive bands. This book provides more than 275 illustrated exercises for the therapist, chiropractor, physician, or healthcare professional to photocopy for patient use and formulate into a comprehensive resistive band exercise program.

Exercises were categorized by body position, and listed by both their common and technical names. The **Purpose** of the exercises and the **Instructions** were written in laymen's terms. Each page includes a **Special Protocols/Notes** section to enable the healthcare professional to modify the exercise and customize each patient program.

Case Studies and **Treatment Protocols** using resistive bands provide the clinician with examples of how to integrate resistive bands into a treatment regimen. The **Electromyography Study,** using five of the resistive band exercises from this book, was included to help identify the intensity of specific muscles firing during a given exercise.

I hope the exercises presented in this book help augment each clinician's repertoire of exercises using resistive bands. Furthermore, I encourage each clinician to create new exercises using Swiss balls, foam rollers, and balance boards in conjunction with resistive bands, to help facilitate the individual needs of their patients.

CAROLINE CORNING CREAGER, P.T.

Table of Contents

CHAPTER ONE

Principles and Concepts of Resistive Bands

Introduction

Brightly colored resistive bands have adorned the walls, floors, and doors of health clubs, and therapy, chiropractic, and physician clinics throughout the world since the 1970s. Currently, thousands, if not millions of people, use resistive bands in their daily workout routines. This rapid rise in resistive band popularity may be attributed to the band's simplicity.

A resistive band — an elastic strip or tube of rubber material — is lightweight, portable, inexpensive, versatile, and offers variable resistance. Many patient populations, (cardiac, chronic pain, geriatric, neurologic, orthopedic, pediatric, prenatal and post-partum, sports medicine, and world-class athletes), use the bands in a variety of positions to simulate sport-specific exercises, activities of daily living, and/or work-related strengthening positions.

Resistive bands, also commonly known as elastic bands, exercise bands, elastic tubing, Thera-Bands®, Dyna-Bands™, or Rep Bands™ are designed to introduce progressive resistance to an exercise program. The different color-coded resistance levels allow the healthcare professional to customize strengthening programs to meet the needs of their patients. Hintermeister et al. concluded that the "external load provided by the elastic resistance device allows patients to modify their exercises to match their rehabilitation progress."[1]

Clinical and home-based resistance training programs that use resistive bands are routinely recommended by healthcare professionals. The following research studies indicate the rehabilitative potential of resistive bands.

- Mikesky et al. found that adults over the age of 65 who adhered to a home-based elastic tubing program increased: training resistance by an average of 82%, isokinetic eccentric knee extension strength by 12%, and flexion strength by 10%.[2]

- Mostardi and Chapman's study documented a 9% increase in muscular strength in sedentary women when they used resistive bands.[3]
- Page et al. report that resistive bands are effective in increasing eccentric force production by 19.8% in the posterior rotator cuff of a pitching shoulder.[4]
- Research by Topp et al. suggests "older adults may realize reduced gait velocities and improved measures of dynamic balance, and may maintain or improve measures of static balance through strength training," using resistive bands.[5]
- Hintermeister et al. also quantified muscle activation levels, knee-joint angles, and applied force during elastic resistance knee exercises. "The data on muscle activation levels and force of the elastic resistance device support the use of these exercises (single knee dip, double knee dip, leg press, hamstring pull, and side-to-side jump) in a progressive, functional rehabilitation program."[6]

Resistive band exercises can add diversification to treatment regimens and appeal to all ages and patient populations. As research has shown, using resistive bands improves strength and balance; and patients readily participate because it is so simple, inexpensive, lightweight, portable, and very versatile. This is why resistive bands have been so successful and popular in the clinic, workplace, home, and clubs.

RESISTIVE BAND SIZES

Resistive bands are usually sold in rolls of 6-yard lengths (5.5 m) and 50-yard lengths (45.8 m) that are 6 inches (15 cm) wide, and so may be customized to any length. Resistive band length is determined by patient height, exercise position, and/or goal of the exercise. For most exercises in this book, a 4-foot length (3.7 m) of resistive band was used.

Begin patients on a low band resistance and progressively

increase the resistance level as strength improves. Resistive bands are color-coded — a visual cue to both the patient and the practitioner as to what resistive band level is being used.

To make exercises more difficult, shorten the length of band or double the band into a loop. To make exercises easier, use a longer piece of band.

The Hygenic Corporation has determined the pounds (newtons) of pull required to stretch single lengths and loops of Thera-Bands ranging in lengths from 14 inches (35 cm) to 36 inches (90 cm). Please refer to **Pounds (Newtons) of Pull Required to Stretch a Single Length or Loop of Resistive Band (Thera-Band)** on page 5.

For additional information, please refer patients to the **Resistive Band Exercise Suggestions** on page 6 and **Knot-Tying Techniques for Resistive Band** on page 7.

RESISTIVE BAND STRIPS

Resistive band strips can be made from resistive band rolls. To make resistive band strips, take a piece of 6-inch-wide (15cm) resistive band and cut ¼-inch (.64cm) strips from the band.

The length of resistive band strips is also determined by exercise position and/or goal of the exercise. A 4- to 6-inch (10–15cm) strip of resistive band was used for most of the hand exercises in this book.

RESISTIVE PUTTY AND BALLS

Resistive putty is similar to resistive bands in that it is also color-coded to illustrate the level of resistance being used. Begin patients on a low resistance and progressively increase the level as their strength improves.

Several different balls and sizes are used in this book. A 55 or 65 cm vinyl ball is used for sitting and standing exercises, and a

20 cm foam ball is used for exercises that require a ball between the knees.

Pounds (Newtons) of Pull
Required to Stretch a Single Length or Loop
of Resistive Band (Thera-Band®)

Reprinted with permission from the Hygenic Corporation

The following tables show the pounds of pull required to stretch a single length or a loop of Thera-Band Resistive Exerciser to various lengths. Pulls were measured using a pull-spring scale.

SINGLE LENGTH   (starting length of 6" W x 12" L band)

U.S.	Pull in pounds for various weights or thicknesses							
Extended Length (inches)	Tan Extra Thin	Yellow Thin	Red Medium	Green Heavy	Blue Extra Heavy	Black Special Heavy	Silver Super Heavy	Gold Max
14	.500	.75	1.00	1.25	1.50	2.00	5.00	7.20
16	1.00	1.50	2.00	2.50	3.00	4.00	9.00	11.20
20	1.50	2.25	3.50	4.25	6.25	7.50	12.00	16.20
24	2.00	2.50	4.50	5.00	7.50	9.00	15.00	20.70
28	2.50	3.00	5.50	6.00	9.00	10.00	17.50	24.30
32	2.70	3.50	6.50	7.00	10.25	11.25	20.00	27.70
36	3.00	4.00	7.50	8.00	12.00	13.00	23.00	30.60

Metric	Pull in newtons for various weights or thicknesses							
Extended Length (centimeters)	Tan Extra Thin	Yellow Thin	Red Medium	Green Heavy	Blue Extra Heavy	Black Special Heavy	Silver Super Heavy	Gold Max
35	2.25	3.25	4.50	5.50	6.50	9.00	22.25	32.00
40	4.50	6.75	9.00	11.00	13.25	17.75	40.00	49.75
50	6.75	10.00	15.50	19.00	27.75	33.25	53.50	72.00
60	9.00	11.00	20.00	22.25	33.25	40.00	66.75	92.00
70	11.00	13.25	24.50	26.75	40.00	44.50	77.25	108.00
80	12.00	15.50	29.00	31.25	45.50	50.00	89.00	123.25
90	13.25	17.75	33.25	35.50	53.50	57.75	102.25	136.00

LOOP   (starting length of loop 12")

U.S.	Pull in pounds for various weights or thicknesses							
Extended Length (inches)	Tan Extra Thin	Yellow Thin	Red Medium	Green Heavy	Blue Extra Heavy	Black Special Heavy	Silver Super Heavy	Gold Max
14	1.00	1.50	2.00	2.50	3.00	4.00	10.00	14.40
16	1.50	3.00	4.00	5.00	6.00	8.00	18.00	22.40
20	3.00	4.50	7.00	8.50	12.50	15.00	24.00	32.40
24	4.10	5.00	9.00	10.00	15.00	18.00	30.00	41.40
28	4.50	6.00	11.00	12.00	18.00	20.00	35.00	48.60
32	5.50	7.00	13.00	14.00	20.50	22.50	40.00	55.40
36	6.00	8.00	15.00	16.00	24.00	26.00	46.00	61.20

Metric	Pull in newtons for various weights or thicknesses							
Extended Length (centimeters)	Tan Extra Thin	Yellow Thin	Red Medium	Green Heavy	Blue Extra Heavy	Black Special Heavy	Silver Super Heavy	Gold Max
35	4.50	6.75	9.00	11.00	13.25	17.75	44.50	64.00
40	6.75	13.25	17.75	22.25	26.75	35.50	80.00	99.50
50	13.25	20.00	31.25	37.75	55.50	66.75	106.75	144.00
60	18.25	22.50	40.00	44.50	66.75	80.00	133.50	184.00
70	20.00	26.75	49.00	53.50	80.00	89.00	155.75	216.00
80	24.50	31.25	57.75	62.25	91.25	100.00	178.00	246.50
90	26.75	35.50	66.75	71.25	106.75	115.75	204.50	272.25

Resistive Band Exercise Suggestions

PURPOSE: To use resistive bands in a safe and effective manner.

1. Always examine resistive bands for flaws, tears, or brittleness to prevent bands from breaking or tearing while exercising.
2. Tie a safe and secure knot in the resistive band to keep it from slipping. Please refer to Knot-Tying Techniques for Resistive Bands, page 7.
3. Do not hold your breath while exercising. Exhale as band becomes taunt. Inhale when band relaxes.
4. Do exercises slowly and rhythmically. Do not allow the band to snap back.
5. Maintain good posture while exercising with the resistive band. Follow the instructions as indicated on exercise page, unless otherwise directed by a healthcare professional.
6. Begin using a low band resistance and progressively increase the level of resistance as strength improves.
7. To make exercises more difficult, shorten the length of the band or double the band forming a loop.
8. To make exercises easier, use a longer piece of band.
9. Prevent the band from pulling on leg or body hair by wearing long pants or a long-sleeved shirt.
10. Store resistive bands in a dark, cool area (21°C/ 70°F) to increase the life of the bands.

SPECIAL PROTOCOLS/NOTES: _____

_____

_____

_____

PATIENT NAME: _____ DATE: _____

THERAPIST NAME: _____

Knot-Tying Techniques for Resistive Bands

PURPOSE: To tie a safe and secure figure-eight knot in a resistive band.

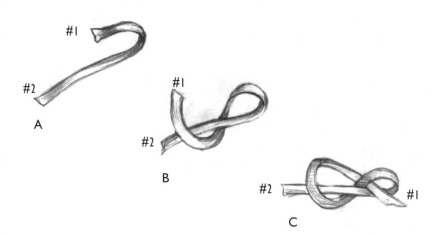

INSTRUCTION:
1. To tie a figure-eight knot in a resistive band, slip end of band (#1) underneath opposite side of band (#2) (illustration A).

2. Pull end #1 up and over opposite side #2 (illustration B).

3. Pull end #1 under and through top loop (illustration C).

4. Tighten knot by pulling on both ends of band.

SPECIAL PROTOCOLS/NOTES: _____
_____
_____
_____

PATIENT NAME: _____ DATE: _____

THERAPIST NAME: _____

Protocols for Using Resistive Bands

INDICATIONS
1. decreased range of motion
2. decreased strength
3. decreased endurance
4. decreased proprioception
5. decreased neural flexibility
6. decreased coordination
7. decreased visual tracking
8. decreased kinesthetic awareness

PRECAUTIONS
1. muscular fatigue
2. cardiovascular fatigue
   a. shortness of breath
   b. light-headedness
   c. pallor
   d. nausea
   e. angina
3. adhering to weight restrictions (i.e., non-weight bearing, partial weight bearing, etc.)
4. following specific injury precautions (i.e., do not exceed 45 degrees of external rotation four weeks' status post rotator cuff repair)
5. superseding patient tolerance level
6. recognizing signs of sensory overload
   a. pupil dilation
   b. sweaty palms
   c. changes in respiration rate
   d. flushing or pallor
   e. complaints of dizziness
7. wrapping a resistive band around an appendage too tightly may impede circulation
8. tying a knot incorrectly may cause the resistive band to slip or untie

9. slipping of a resistive band on an area covered with hair may cause discomfort
10. snapping bands at one another may be harmful
11. recognizing signs of latex sensitivity
    a. rash, redness or swelling on skin, 6–48 hours after contact with latex band
    b. eczema
    c. itching
    d. hay fever like symptoms
    e. wheezing
    f. angioedema of eyes and lips
    g. anaphylactic shock

CONTRAINDICATIONS
1. increased pain
2. dizziness/nausea
3. exercising with a flawed, torn or brittle resistive band
4. providing latex resistive band to a patient with latex sensitivity
5. using resistive bands inappropriately, i.e., snapping bands at other people

Treatment Protocols with Resistive Bands

The following information is designed to help the clinician become acquainted with using resistive bands in a treatment situation. Each individual patient is unique and may vary from the criterion presented below. Please use good judgment and common sense when applying this information to your patients. Use the following information only as a reference guide to your treatments; observe the patient's signs and symptoms, then carefully and methodically apply your own skills to effect a positive treatment outcome.[8]

CARPAL TUNNEL SYNDROME

Carpal tunnel may present as a result of one or more of the following: repetitive motion, trauma, pregnancy, and collagen disease. The median nerve travels through the carpal tunnel and becomes compressed with inflammation or narrowing of the carpal tunnel itself. Identify any source from work or home environment that may be causing the patient to repeat the same motions and reduce or eliminate this motion from their routine. Reduce inflammation using the appropriate modalities. Instruct the patient in soft tissue mobilization, and gentle stretching and strengthening exercises.

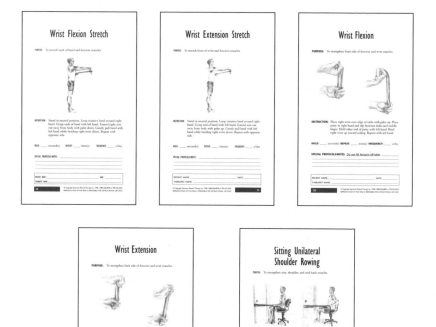

LATERAL EPICONDYLITIS

Lateral Epicondylitis usually affects the dominant arm of adults between the ages of 20 and 50 years old. Inflammation and pain is generally located over the lateral epicondylar region. Reduce inflammation using the appropriate modality. Evaluate and modify the patient's workplace or athletic equipment. Instruct the patient in stretching and strengthening exercises for the forearm extensors, especially the extensor carpi radialis brevis and extensor digitorum muscles. These muscle are famous for contributing to lateral epicondylitis.

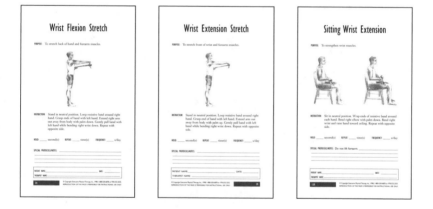

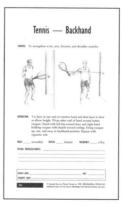

ROTATOR CUFF TEAR

The rotator cuff is made up of four muscles: the supraspinatus, infraspinatus, teres minor, and subscapularis. The supraspinatus muscle is most commonly ruptured, especially at its insertion. Follow postsurgical precautions and contraindications. When appropriate progress has been made, graduate the patient from passive to active assistive and to active range-of-motion and strengthening exercises.

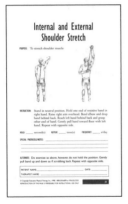

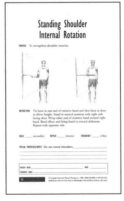

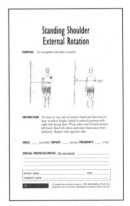

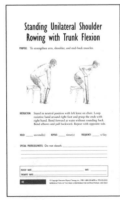

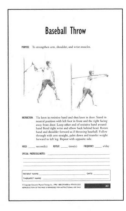

CERVICAL STRAIN/WHIPLASH

Cervical strain or whiplash is a common consequence of a motor vehicle accident. Initially, pain and swelling may be prevalent in the cervical region. Mobilize the soft tissue when indicated and apply the appropriate modality to reduce swelling. At times when symptoms are acute, try strengthening the patient's cervical region indirectly, i.e., try a supine hip hike exercise as illustrated below to provide indirect range of motion and strengthening of the scalenes and sternocleidomastoid muscles. Progress to direct range-of-motion and strengthening exercises.

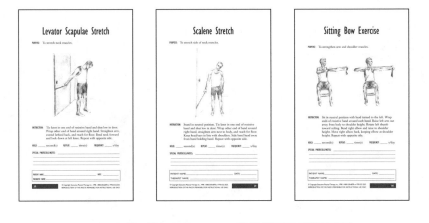

LOW BACK PAIN

More than 80 percent of the population experiences low back pain at some time in their life. Lumbar strain, facet dysfunction, and herniated discs can all contribute to low back pain. Evaluate the patient and determine the etiology of low back pain. If inflammation is prevalent, apply the appropriate modality to the region to reduce swelling. If indicated, instruct the patient in thoracic, lumbar, and lower extremity stretches. Progress to abdominal and lumbar strengthening exercises.

Hamstring and Gastrocnemius Stretch

PURPOSE: To stretch back of thigh muscles.

INSTRUCTION: Lie on back. Bend right knee toward chest and wrap resistive band around right foot. Straighten knee. Gently pull band toward body, pointing toes down toward nose. Keep knee as straight as possible. Repeat with opposite side.

HOLD: _____ second(s)   REPEAT: _____ time(s)   FREQUENCY: _____ x/day

SPECIAL PROTOCOLS/NOTES: Do not lift head from floor.

PATIENT NAME: _____ DATE: _____
THERAPIST NAME: _____

© Copyright Executive Physical Therapy, Inc., 1998. 1-800-530-6878 or 970-532-3532.
REPRODUCTION OF THIS PAGE IS PERMISSIBLE FOR INSTRUCTIONAL USE ONLY

Sitting Trunk Extension

PURPOSE: To strengthen back and neck muscles.

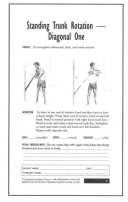

INSTRUCTION: Tie ends of resistive band together and shut knot in door. Sit in chair in neutral position facing door. Loop resistive band around chest. Lean backward keeping back straight. Return to starting position.

HOLD: _____ second(s)   REPEAT: _____ time(s)   FREQUENCY: _____ x/day

SPECIAL PROTOCOLS/NOTES: Do not slouch. _____

PATIENT NAME: _____ DATE: _____
THERAPIST NAME: _____

© Copyright Executive Physical Therapy, Inc., 1998. 1-800-530-6878 or 970-532-3532.
REPRODUCTION OF THIS PAGE IS PERMISSIBLE FOR INSTRUCTIONAL USE ONLY

Standing Trunk Rotation — Diagonal One

PURPOSE: To strengthen abdominal, back, and trunk muscles.

INSTRUCTION: Tie knot in one end of resistive band and shut knot in door at knee height. Wrap other end of resistive band around left hand. Stand in neutral position with right hip toward door. Bend at waist and rotate trunk toward right hip. Straighten at waist and rotate trunk and head over left shoulder. Repeat with opposite side.

HOLD: _____ second(s)   REPEAT: _____ time(s)   FREQUENCY: _____ x/day

SPECIAL PROTOCOLS/NOTES: Do not rotate hips with upper body. Keep hips facing forward and arms close to body. _____

PATIENT NAME: _____ DATE: _____
THERAPIST NAME: _____

© Copyright Executive Physical Therapy, Inc., 1998. 1-800-530-6878 or 970-532-3532.
REPRODUCTION OF THIS PAGE IS PERMISSIBLE FOR INSTRUCTIONAL USE ONLY

Prone Trunk Rotation on Ball

PURPOSE: To strengthen arm, bid back, and shoulder muscles. To improve trunk flexibility.

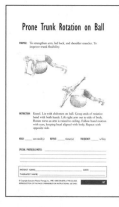

INSTRUCTION: Kneel. Lie with abdomen on ball. Grasp ends of resistive band with both hands. Lift right arm out to side of body. Rotate torso as arm is raised to ceiling. Follow hand motion with eyes, keeping head aligned with body. Repeat with opposite side.

HOLD: _____ second(s)   REPEAT: _____ time(s)   FREQUENCY: _____ x/day

SPECIAL PROTOCOLS/NOTES: _____

PATIENT NAME: _____ DATE: _____
THERAPIST NAME: _____

© Copyright Executive Physical Therapy, Inc., 1998. 1-800-530-6878 or 970-532-3532.
REPRODUCTION OF THIS PAGE IS PERMISSIBLE FOR INSTRUCTIONAL USE ONLY

Supine Lower Abdominal Reverse Curle

PURPOSE: To strengthen lower abdominal muscles.

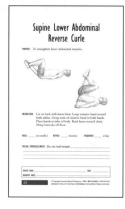

INSTRUCTION: Lie on back with knees bent. Loop resistive band around both ankles. Grasp ends of resistive band in both hands. Place hands at sides of body. Bend knees toward chest, lifting buttocks off floor.

HOLD: _____ second(s)   REPEAT: _____ time(s)   FREQUENCY: _____ x/day

SPECIAL PROTOCOLS/NOTES: Do not hold breath. _____

PATIENT NAME: _____ DATE: _____
THERAPIST NAME: _____

© Copyright Executive Physical Therapy, Inc., 1998. 1-800-530-6878 or 970-532-3532.
REPRODUCTION OF THIS PAGE IS PERMISSIBLE FOR INSTRUCTIONAL USE ONLY

PIRIFORMIS SYNDROME

The piriformis muscle is an external rotator of the hip, and abductor of the hip when the knee is flexed. The sciatic nerve may run superior to, inferior to, or through the middle of the piriformis muscle. The piriformis muscle may become inflamed, tight, and painful. If inflammation exists, apply the appropriate modality to the piriformis area to reduce swelling. Administer soft tissue mobilization to piriformis muscle and instruct the patient in stretching and strengthening exercises.

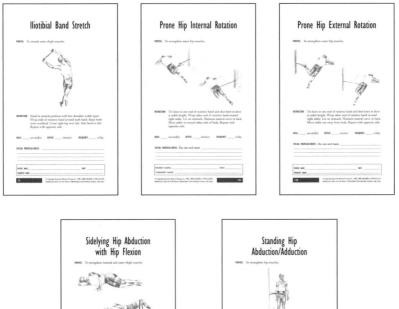

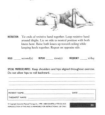

PATELLOFEMORAL DYSFUNCTION

   Patellofemoral dysfunction may be caused by one or more of the following: misalignment of the patella due to weakness of the vastus medialis oblique, or tightness of the iliotibial band/gluteus medius muscle. Evaluate the patient to determine the cause of the patellofemoral dysfunction. If indicated, instruct the patient in stretching exercises for the hamstrings, quadriceps, gluteus medius, and/or iliotibial band; and strengthening exercises for the vastus medialis oblique muscle. Progress the patient through muscle reeducation exercises so that the increased length and strength of the muscle helps the body to internalize a "normal" pattern of movement.

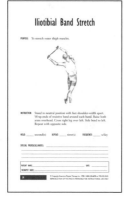

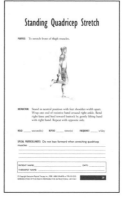

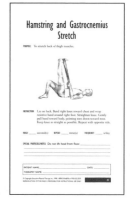

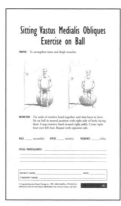

ANKLE SPRAIN

The anterior talofibular ligament is the most commonly injured ligament with ankle sprains, caused by an excessive inversion stress of the foot. Symptoms include pain, swelling, and limited ankle range of motion. Begin by administering R.I.C.E. instructions: Rest, Ice (within 24 hours of injury), Compression, and Elevation. Instruct patient in gentle non-weight-bearing range-of-motion exercises and progress to weight-bearing range-of-motion exercises and strengthening.

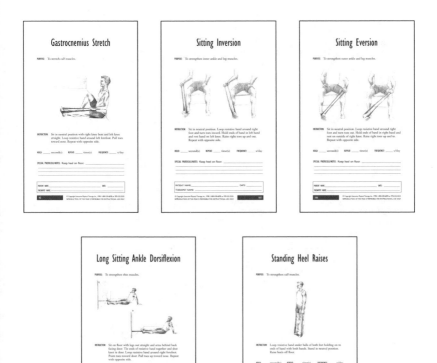

CEREBROVASCULAR ACCIDENT

A cerebrovascular accident or "stroke" results when the blood supply to the brain is restricted. Multiple deficits can occur that affect motor function, sensation, mental status, perception, and language skills. Motor loss is often described as hemiplegia that occurs on the side of the body opposite the site of the lesion. Treatment for motor loss can include muscle reeducation, facilitation, positioning, and abnormal postural corrections. Treatment should focus on the areas of deficit with emphasis on normalizing both function and quality of life.

Supine Shoulder Protraction

PURPOSE: To strengthen shoulder muscles.

INSTRUCTION: Wrap ends of resistive band around each hand. Loop hand behind back. Lie on back in neutral position with knees bent. Bend elbows and push hands toward ceiling.

HOLD: _____ second(s)   REPEAT: _____ time(s)   FREQUENCY: _____ x/day

SPECIAL PROTOCOL/NOTES: Do not round shoulders. _____

VARIATION: Follow instructions as above, however, push only one hand toward ceiling at a time.

PATIENT NAME: _____ DATE: _____
THERAPIST NAME: _____

Sidelying Hip Flexion in Bed

PURPOSE: To strengthen front of thigh muscles.

INSTRUCTION: Tie both ends of resistive band to bed rail. Lie on side in bed in neutral position facing away from bed rail. Loop resistive band below knee. Straighten top leg and place behind bottom leg. Move leg forward. Repeat on opposite side.

HOLD: _____ second(s)   REPEAT: _____ time(s)   FREQUENCY: _____ x/day

SPECIAL PROTOCOL/NOTES: Keep shoulders and hips aligned throughout exercise. Do not allow hips to roll forward or backward.

PATIENT NAME: _____ DATE: _____
THERAPIST NAME: _____

Sidelying Hip Extension in Bed

PURPOSE: To strengthen back of thigh muscles.

INSTRUCTION: Tie both ends of resistive band to bed rail. Lie on side in bed in neutral position facing bed rail. Loop resistive band around top knee. Straighten top leg and place in front of bottom leg. Move leg backward. Repeat on opposite side.

HOLD: _____ second(s)   REPEAT: _____ time(s)   FREQUENCY: _____ x/day

SPECIAL PROTOCOL/NOTES: Keep shoulders and hips aligned throughout exercise. Do not allow hips to roll forward or backward.

PATIENT NAME: _____ DATE: _____
THERAPIST NAME: _____

Sitting Knee Flexion

PURPOSE: To strengthen back of thigh muscles.

INSTRUCTION: Tie ends of resistive band together and shut knot in door. Loop band around right ankle. Sit in chair in neutral position facing door with right knee straight. Bend knee back toward chair. Repeat with opposite side.

HOLD: _____ second(s)   REPEAT: _____ time(s)   FREQUENCY: _____ x/day

SPECIAL PROTOCOL/NOTES: _____

PATIENT NAME: _____ DATE: _____
THERAPIST NAME: _____

Sitting Knee Extension

PURPOSE: To strengthen front of thigh muscles.

INSTRUCTION: Sit in chair in neutral position. Tie resistive band around right chair leg and loop around right ankle. Straighten knee. Repeat with opposite side.

HOLD: _____ second(s)   REPEAT: _____ time(s)   FREQUENCY: _____ x/day

SPECIAL PROTOCOL/NOTES: _____

PATIENT NAME: _____ DATE: _____
THERAPIST NAME: _____

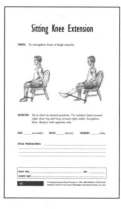

Multiple Sclerosis

Multiple sclerosis is a demyelinating disease of the central nervous system. It mostly affects young adults and can often present with fluctuating periods of remission and exacerbation. Clinical features of multiple sclerosis include spasticity, impaired motor function, ataxia, intention tremors, impaired sensation, visual deficits, speech problems, and bowel and bladder dysfunction. Evaluate to determine the deficit areas. Treatment focus should be to improve or at least maintain strength, motor control, coordination, gait, activities of daily living, sensory feedback, and range of motion to all joints. Treatment is most often long-term and should include an ongoing program for the patient to continue to perform at home.

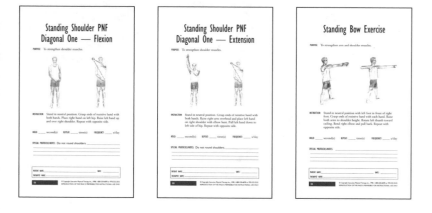

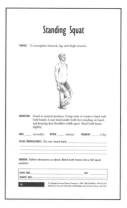

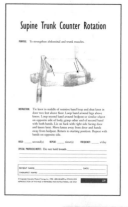

PARKINSON'S DISEASE

Parkinson's disease is a chronic progressive disease of the nervous system involving the basal ganglia. Onset usually occurs after the age of 50. Posture, balance, and gait are most commonly affected by Parkinson's disease. Treatment should focus on promoting improved posture; functional strength and range of motion in the neck, trunk, and extremities; and improving functional mobility for balance and gait.

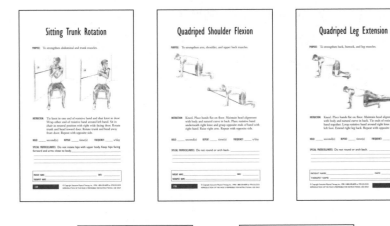

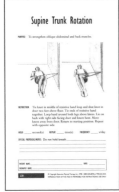

LATEX ALLERGIES

A latex allergy develops after repetitive or prolonged exposure to latex products or airborne latex antigenic proteins. In addition, the antigenic proteins must gain entry into the body. Latex proteins generally traverse the skin's barrier via a cut, lesion, or other form of skin breakdown. "The proteins in the latex itself appear to be the primary source of the allergic reactions."[9]

Cumulative exposure to latex products can cause allergic reactions to worsen. Latex allergy symptoms may include: rash, redness or swelling on skin, 6–48 hours after contact with latex product, eczema, itching, hay fever like symptoms (runny nose, sneezing, itchy/watery eyes), difficulty breathing, wheezing, coughing, angioedema of eyes and lips, and in the worst-case scenario, anaphylactic shock.

"An estimated 7% to 20% of health care providers today are at risk from exposure to latex medical supplies and latex gloves."[10] Individuals at risk are "frequently exposed to latex, have had several surgeries and hospitalizations that have exposed (them) to latex, or if (they) are allergic to certain foods including, avocado, banana, celery, chestnuts, kiwi, papaya, potato, and tomato."[11]

Amazingly, about 40,000 products contain latex. The following is a list of common latex products found at work or in the home: **resistive band**, Leukopore tape (McConnell tape), rubber bands, balloons, chewing gum, erasers, carpet backing, computer mouse pads, electric cords, elastic in clothing, shoe soles, adhesives including envelope and stamp glue, condoms, goggles, catheters, syringes, IV tubing, and stethoscope tubes.

The best way to prevent latex sensitivity is to avoid using latex products. Fortunately for the healthcare community, latex-free resistive bands are now available on the market. The Magister Corporation, and recently the Hygenic Corporation, produce latex-free resistive bands: Rep Bands, and latex-free Thera-Bands, respectively.

In the event a latex resistive band is used in the clinic or at home, thoroughly wash hands (or any other body part coming in contact with the band) with soap and water. Avoid using the band when a break in the skin is detected that is not protected by a bandage. Keep work area free of resistive band powder by dusting off equipment and vacuuming floors.

NOTES

1. Hintermeister, Robert and Bey, Michael, et al. "Quantification of Elastic Resistance Knee Rehabilitation Exercises." *JOSPT* 28(1): 1998, pp. 40–50.
2. Mikesky, Alan and Topp, Robert, et al. "Efficacy of a Home-Based Training Program for Older Adults Using Elastic Tubing," *E J Appl. Physiol. Occup. Physiol.* 69: 1994, pp. 316–320.
3. Mostardi, Richard and Chapman, Elizabeth. "Improvement in Muscular Strength with The Use of Wide Width Therapeutic Resistive Bands." Akron City Hospital and The University of Akron.
4. Page, Philip and Lamberth, John, et al. "Posterior Rotator Cuff Strengthening Using Thera-Band in a Functional Diagonal Pattern in Collegiate Baseball Pitchers," *Athletic Training, NATA* 28(4): 1993, pp. 346–354.
5. Topp, Robert and Mikesky, Alan, et al. " The Effect of a 12-week Dynamic Resistance Strength Training Program on Gait Velocity and Balance of Older Adults," *Gerontol.* 33(4): 1993, pp. 501–506.
6. Hintermeister, p. 45.
7. Hygenic Corporation. *Thera-Band System of Progressive Resistance, Instruction Manual,* 3rd Edition. (Akron, OH: The Hygenic Corporation, 1996).
8. Maitland, G.D. *Vertebral Manipulation,* 5th Edition. (Butterworth & Co. Ltd., 1986).
9. Lockard, Joanne. "Living with a Latex Allergy," *PT Magazine,* March 1998, pp. 36–42.
10. Ibid.
11. "Are You Allergic to Latex?" *Safety+Health,* May 1998, p. 63.

Stretching Exercises

CHAPTER TWO

Stretching Techniques

PURPOSE: To safely and effectively increase muscle length.

INSTRUCTIONS: 1. Avoid bouncing.

2. Slowly stretch into level of tolerance, not pain.

3. Do not hold your breath.

4. Repeat stretch three to five times.

5. Repeat on both sides of body.

SPECIAL PROTOCOLS/NOTES: _____

_____

_____

_____

PATIENT NAME: _____ DATE: _____

THERAPIST NAME: _____

Cervical Stretch

PURPOSE: To stretch neck muscles.

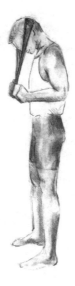

INSTRUCTION: Stand in neutral position. Hold ends of resistive band in each hand. Loop band behind head. Gently pull band down while lowering chin toward chest.

HOLD: _____ second(s) **REPEAT:** _____ time(s) **FREQUENCY:** _____ x/day

SPECIAL PROTOCOLS/NOTES: _____
_____
_____
_____

PATIENT NAME: _____   DATE: _____

THERAPIST NAME: _____

Scalene Stretch

PURPOSE: To stretch side of neck muscles.

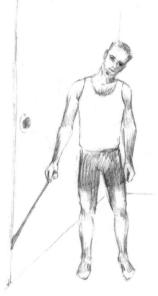

INSTRUCTION: Stand in neutral position. Tie knot in one end of resistive band and shut low in door. Wrap other end of band around right hand, straighten arm next to body, and reach for floor. Keep head/ears in line with shoulders. Side bend head away from hand holding band. Repeat with opposite side.

HOLD: _____ second(s) **REPEAT:** _____ time(s) **FREQUENCY:** _____ x/day

SPECIAL PROTOCOLS/NOTES: _____

_____

_____

_____

PATIENT NAME: _____ DATE: _____

THERAPIST NAME: _____

Levator Scapulae Stretch

PURPOSE: To stretch neck muscles.

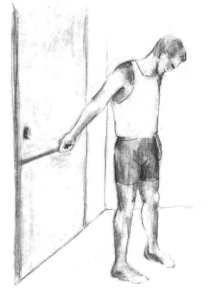

INSTRUCTION: Tie knot in one end of resistive band and shut knot low in door. Wrap other end of band around right hand. Straighten arm, extend behind back, and reach for floor. Bend neck forward and look down at left knee. Repeat with opposite side.

HOLD: _____ second(s) **REPEAT:** _____ time(s) **FREQUENCY:** _____ x/day

SPECIAL PROTOCOLS/NOTES: _____
_____
_____
_____

PATIENT NAME: _____ DATE: _____
THERAPIST NAME: _____

Internal and External Shoulder Stretch

PURPOSE: To stretch shoulder muscles.

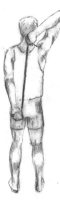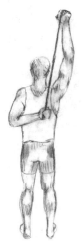

INSTRUCTION: Stand in neutral position. Hold one end of resistive band in right hand. Raise right arm overhead. Bend elbow and drop band behind back. Reach left hand behind back and grasp other end of band. Gently pull band toward floor with left hand. Raise right arm and gently pull band up toward ceiling with right hand. Repeat with opposite side.

HOLD: _____ second(s) **REPEAT:** _____ time(s) **FREQUENCY:** _____ x/day

SPECIAL PROTOCOLS/NOTES: _____
_____
_____

ALTERNATE: Do exercise as above, however, do not hold the position. Gently pull band up and down as if scrubbing back. Repeat with opposite side.

PATIENT NAME: _____   DATE: _____

THERAPIST NAME: _____

Deltoid Stretch

PURPOSE: To stretch shoulder muscles.

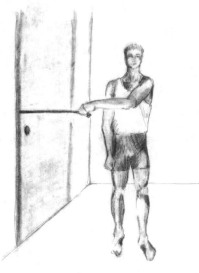

INSTRUCTION: Tie knot in one end of resistive band and shut knot in door. Wrap other end of band around left hand. Straighten left arm across body. Take side steps to left until stretch is felt in left shoulder. Repeat with opposite side.

HOLD: _____ second(s) **REPEAT:** _____ time(s) **FREQUENCY:** _____ x/day

SPECIAL PROTOCOLS/NOTES: _____

_____

_____

_____

PATIENT NAME: _____ DATE: _____

THERAPIST NAME: _____

Tricep Stretch

PURPOSE: To stretch back of arm muscles.

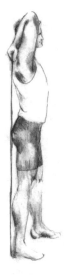

INSTRUCTION: Stand in neutral position. Wrap one end of band around right hand. Raise arm overhead and bend elbow. Lower other end of band behind back to floor with elbow bent. Step on band to take up any slack. Repeat with opposite side.

HOLD: _____ second(s) **REPEAT:** _____ time(s) **FREQUENCY:** _____ x/day

SPECIAL PROTOCOLS/NOTES: _____
_____
_____
_____

PATIENT NAME: _____ DATE: _____

THERAPIST NAME: _____

Wrist Flexion Stretch

PURPOSE: To stretch back of hand and forearm muscles.

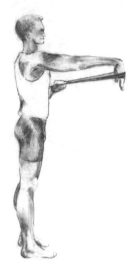

INSTRUCTION: Stand in neutral position. Grasp ends of resistive band with left hand. Loop band around right hand. Extend right arm out away from body with palm down. Gently pull band with left hand while bending right wrist down. Repeat with opposite side.

HOLD: _____ second(s) **REPEAT:** _____ time(s) **FREQUENCY:** _____ x/day

SPECIAL PROTOCOLS/NOTES: _____
_____
_____
_____

PATIENT NAME: _____ DATE: _____
THERAPIST NAME: _____

Wrist Extension Stretch

PURPOSE: To stretch front of wrist and forearm muscles.

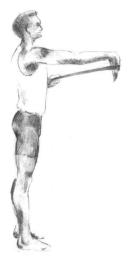

INSTRUCTION: Stand in neutral position. Grasp ends of resistive band with left hand. Loop band around right hand. Extend arm out away from body with palm up. Gently pull band with left hand while bending right wrist down. Repeat with opposite side.

HOLD: _____ second(s) **REPEAT:** _____ time(s) **FREQUENCY:** _____ x/day

SPECIAL PROTOCOLS/NOTES: _____

_____

_____

_____

PATIENT NAME: _____   DATE: _____

THERAPIST NAME: _____

Pectoralis Stretch

PURPOSE: To stretch chest muscles.

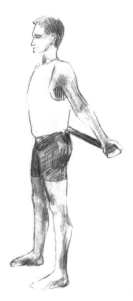

INSTRUCTION: Stand in neutral position. Wrap ends of resistive band around each hand. Raise both arms overhead. Lower hands down toward floor, keeping palms facing forward.

HOLD: _____ second(s) **REPEAT:** _____ time(s) **FREQUENCY:** _____ x/day

SPECIAL PROTOCOLS/NOTES: _____

_____

_____

_____

PATIENT NAME: _____ DATE: _____

THERAPIST NAME: _____

Side Stretch

PURPOSE: To stretch side of trunk muscles.

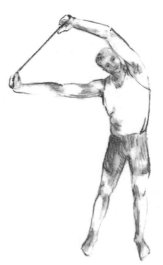

INSTRUCTION: Stand in neutral position with feet shoulder-width apart. Wrap ends of resistive band around each hand. Raise both arms overhead. Side bend to right side. Repeat with opposite side.

HOLD: _____ second(s) **REPEAT:** _____ time(s) **FREQUENCY:** _____ x/day

SPECIAL PROTOCOLS/NOTES: _____
_____
_____
_____

PATIENT NAME: _____ DATE: _____
THERAPIST NAME: _____

Iliotibial Band Stretch

PURPOSE: To stretch outer thigh muscles.

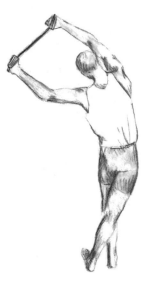

INSTRUCTION: Stand in neutral position with feet shoulder-width apart. Wrap ends of resistive band around each hand. Raise both arms overhead. Cross left leg over right. Side bend to left. Repeat with opposite side.

HOLD: _____ second(s) **REPEAT:** _____ time(s) **FREQUENCY:** _____ x/day

SPECIAL PROTOCOLS/NOTES: _____

_____

_____

_____

PATIENT NAME: _____ DATE: _____

THERAPIST NAME: _____

Standing Quadricep Stretch

PURPOSE: To stretch front of thigh muscles.

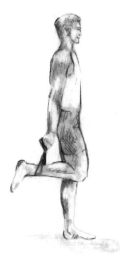

INSTRUCTION: Stand in neutral position with feet shoulder-width apart. Wrap one end of resistive band around right ankle. Bend right knee and heel toward buttock by gently lifting band with right hand. Repeat with opposite side.

HOLD: _____ second(s) **REPEAT:** _____ time(s) **FREQUENCY:** _____ x/day

SPECIAL PROTOCOLS/NOTES: Do not lean forward when stretching quadricep muscles. _____

_____

_____

PATIENT NAME: _____ DATE: _____

THERAPIST NAME: _____

Prone Quadricep Stretch

PURPOSE: To stretch front of thigh muscles.

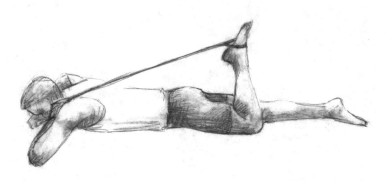

INSTRUCTION: Lie on stomach in neutral position. Loop resistive band around left ankle and grasp other end of band with left hand. Bend left knee. Gently pull ankle toward buttock. Repeat with opposite side.

HOLD: _____ second(s) **REPEAT:** _____ time(s) **FREQUENCY:** _____ x/day

SPECIAL PROTOCOLS/NOTES: _____

_____

_____

_____

PATIENT NAME: _____ DATE: _____

THERAPIST NAME: _____

Hamstring and Gastrocnemius Stretch

PURPOSE: To stretch back of thigh muscles.

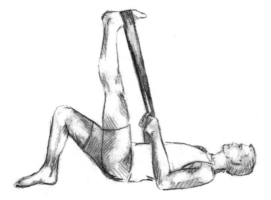

INSTRUCTION: Lie on back. Bend left knee toward chest and loop resistive band around left foot. Straighten knee. Gently pull band toward body, pointing toes down toward nose. Keep knee as straight as possible. Repeat with opposite side.

HOLD: _____ second(s) **REPEAT:** _____ time(s) **FREQUENCY:** _____ x/day

SPECIAL PROTOCOLS/NOTES: Do not lift head from floor. _____

_____

_____

_____

PATIENT NAME: _____ DATE: _____

THERAPIST NAME: _____

Gastrocnemius Stretch

PURPOSE: To stretch calf muscles.

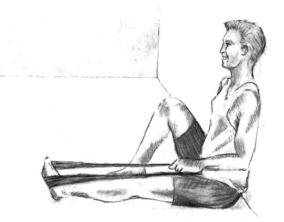

INSTRUCTION: Sit in neutral position with right knee bent and left knee straight. Loop resistive band around left forefoot. Pull toes toward nose. Repeat with opposite side.

HOLD: _____ second(s) **REPEAT:** _____ time(s) **FREQUENCY:** _____ x/day

SPECIAL PROTOCOLS/NOTES: Keep heel on floor. _____
_____
_____
_____

PATIENT NAME: _____	DATE: _____
THERAPIST NAME: _____	

CHAPTER THREE

Standing Exercises

CHAPTER THREE

Standing Neutral Position

PURPOSE: To strengthen muscles in an optimal position to avoid injury.

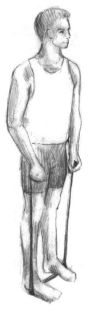

INSTRUCTION: Stand with feet shoulder-width apart. Maintain natural curve in back.

HOLD: _____ second(s) **REPEAT:** _____ time(s) **FREQUENCY:** _____ x/day

SPECIAL PROTOCOLS/NOTES: Do not arch back or slouch. _____

_____

_____

_____

PATIENT NAME: _____ DATE: _____

THERAPIST NAME: _____

Standing Cervical Flexion

PURPOSE: To strengthen front of neck muscles.

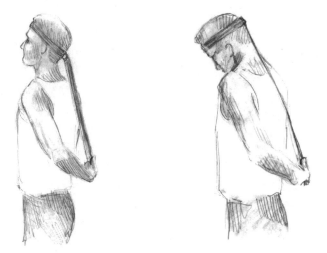

INSTRUCTION: Stand in neutral position with feet shoulder-width apart. Loop resistive band around head and tie knot close to head. Grasp end of band with one hand behind back. Bend head forward. Return head to starting position.

HOLD: _____ second(s) **REPEAT:** _____ time(s) **FREQUENCY:** _____ x/day

SPECIAL PROTOCOLS/NOTES: Do not round shoulders or arch back. _____

_____

_____

_____

PATIENT NAME: _____ DATE: _____

THERAPIST NAME: _____

Standing Cervical Extension

PURPOSE: To strengthen back of neck muscles.

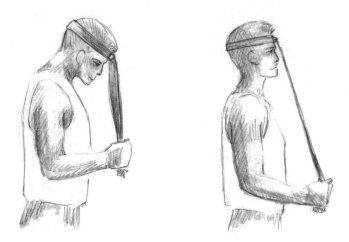

INSTRUCTION: Stand in neutral position with feet shoulder-width apart. Loop resistive band around head and tie knot close to head. Bend head forward. Grasp end of band with one hand. Raise head to starting position.

HOLD: _____ second(s) **REPEAT:** _____ time(s) **FREQUENCY:** _____ x/day

SPECIAL PROTOCOLS/NOTES: Do not round shoulders. _____
_____
_____
_____

PATIENT NAME: _____ DATE: _____
THERAPIST NAME: _____

Standing Cervical Side Bend

PURPOSE: To strengthen side of neck muscles.

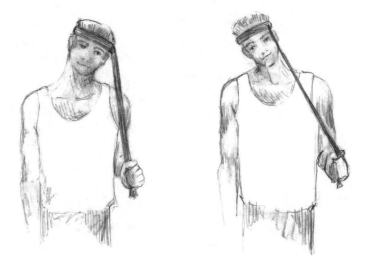

INSTRUCTION: Stand in neutral position with feet shoulder-width apart. Loop resistive band around head and tie knot close to head on left side. Side bend head toward band to the left. Grasp end of band with left hand. Bend head to the right. Repeat with opposite side.

HOLD: _____ second(s) **REPEAT:** _____ time(s) **FREQUENCY:** _____ x/day

SPECIAL PROTOCOLS/NOTES: Do not round shoulders. _____
_____
_____
_____

PATIENT NAME: _____ DATE: _____

THERAPIST NAME: _____

Standing Cervical Rotation

PURPOSE: To strengthen side of neck muscles.

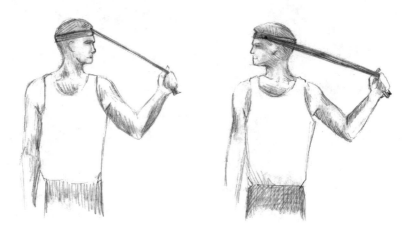

INSTRUCTION: Stand in neutral position with feet shoulder-width apart. Loop resistive band around head and tie knot close to head on left side. Rotate head to the left. Grasp end of band with left hand. Rotate head to the right. Repeat with opposite side.

HOLD: _____ second(s) **REPEAT:** _____ time(s) **FREQUENCY:** _____ x/day

SPECIAL PROTOCOLS/NOTES: Do not round shoulders or arch back.
_____
_____
_____

PATIENT NAME: _____ DATE: _____

THERAPIST NAME: _____

Standing Elbow Flexion

PURPOSE: To strengthen front of arm muscles.

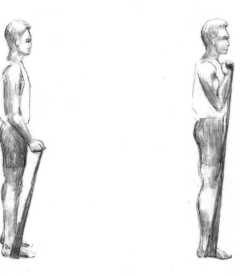

INSTRUCTION: Stand in neutral position with feet shoulder-width apart. Place one end of resistive band under right foot and wrap other end of band around right hand. Bend right elbow. Raise hand toward shoulder. Repeat with opposite side.

HOLD: _____ second(s) **REPEAT:** _____ time(s) **FREQUENCY:** _____ x/day

SPECIAL PROTOCOLS/NOTES: Do not round shoulders. _____
_____
_____
_____

PATIENT NAME: _____   DATE: _____
THERAPIST NAME: _____

Standing Bilateral Elbow Flexion

PURPOSE: To strengthen forearms and front of arm muscles.

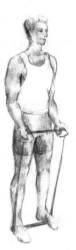 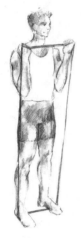

INSTRUCTION: Stand in neutral position with feet shoulder-width apart. Loop resistive band under both feet and grasp ends of band with both hands with palms up. Bend elbows keeping palms up. Raise hands toward shoulders.

HOLD: _____ second(s) **REPEAT:** _____ time(s) **FREQUENCY:** _____ x/day

SPECIAL PROTOCOLS/NOTES: Do not round shoulders. _____
_____
_____
_____

PATIENT NAME: _____ DATE: _____

THERAPIST NAME: _____

Standing Bilateral Elbow Flexion with Palms Down

PURPOSE: To strengthen forearm and front of arm muscles.

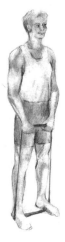 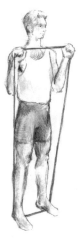

INSTRUCTION: Stand in neutral position with feet shoulder-width apart. Loop resistive band under both feet and grasp ends of band with both hands with palms down. Bend elbows keeping palms down. Raise hands toward shoulders.

HOLD: _____ second(s) **REPEAT:** _____ time(s) **FREQUENCY:** _____ x/day

SPECIAL PROTOCOLS/NOTES: Do not round shoulders.

_____
_____
_____

PATIENT NAME: _____ DATE: _____

THERAPIST NAME: _____

Standing Elbow Extension

PURPOSE: To strengthen back of arm muscles.

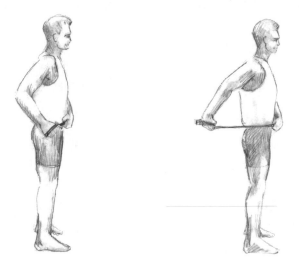

INSTRUCTION: Stand in neutral position. Wrap ends of resistive band around each hand. Place left hand next to right hip. Bend right elbow and place next to side of body. Extend right arm behind back. Repeat with opposite side.

HOLD: _____ second(s) **REPEAT:** _____ time(s) **FREQUENCY:** _____ x/day

SPECIAL PROTOCOLS/NOTES: Do not round shoulders. _____

_____

_____

_____

PATIENT NAME: _____ DATE: _____

THERAPIST NAME: _____

Standing Overhead Elbow Extension

PURPOSE: To strengthen back of arm muscles.

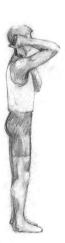 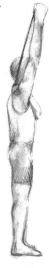

INSTRUCTION: Stand in neutral position. Wrap ends of resistive band around each hand. Place left hand on right shoulder. Raise right arm overhead and bend elbow. Straighten right elbow. Return to starting position. Repeat with opposite side.

HOLD: _____ second(s) **REPEAT:** _____ time(s) **FREQUENCY:** _____ x/day

SPECIAL PROTOCOLS/NOTES: Keep elbow facing forward. Do not allow elbow to drift to side of body.

_____

_____

PATIENT NAME: _____ DATE: _____

THERAPIST NAME: _____

Standing Shoulder Shrugs

PURPOSE: To strengthen shoulder muscles.

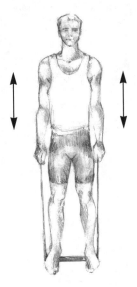

INSTRUCTION: Stand in neutral position. Wrap ends of resistive band around each hand. Loop band under both feet, keeping feet shoulder-width apart. Raise shoulders up toward ears.

HOLD: _____ second(s) **REPEAT:** _____ time(s) **FREQUENCY:** _____ x/day

SPECIAL PROTOCOLS/NOTES: Keep elbows straight. Do not round shoulders.

_____

_____

_____

PATIENT NAME: _____ DATE: _____

THERAPIST NAME: _____

Standing Unilateral Shoulder Flexion

PURPOSE: To strengthen arm and shoulder muscles.

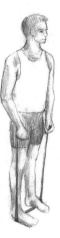 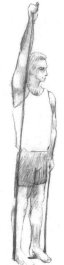

INSTRUCTION: Stand in neutral position with feet shoulder-width apart. Grasp ends of resistive band with both hands. Loop band under both feet. Straighten right elbow. Raise right arm overhead. Repeat with opposite side.

HOLD: _____ second(s) **REPEAT:** _____ time(s) **FREQUENCY:** _____ x/day

SPECIAL PROTOCOLS/NOTES: Do not round shoulders. _____
_____
_____
_____

PATIENT NAME: _____ DATE: _____

THERAPIST NAME: _____

Standing Bilateral Shoulder Flexion

PURPOSE: To strengthen arm and shoulder muscles.

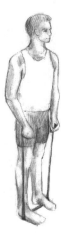 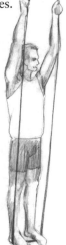

INSTRUCTION: Stand in neutral position with feet shoulder-width apart. Grasp ends of resistive band with both hands. Loop band under both feet. Raise arms overhead.

HOLD: _____ second(s) **REPEAT:** _____ time(s) **FREQUENCY:** _____ x/day

SPECIAL PROTOCOLS/NOTES: Do not round shoulders. _____

_____

_____

_____

PATIENT NAME: _____ DATE: _____

THERAPIST NAME: _____

Standing Upright Row

PURPOSE: To strengthen arm and shoulder muscles.

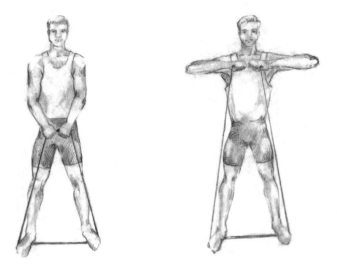

INSTRUCTION: Stand in neutral position with feet shoulder-width apart. Grasp ends of resistive band with both hands. Loop band under both feet. Bring hands together. Raise hands and elbows together to shoulder height.

HOLD: _____ second(s) **REPEAT:** _____ time(s) **FREQUENCY:** _____ x/day

SPECIAL PROTOCOLS/NOTES: Keep elbows and hands in alignment. _____
_____
_____
_____

PATIENT NAME: _____ DATE: _____

THERAPIST NAME: _____

Standing Shoulder Extension

PURPOSE: To strengthen arm and shoulder muscles.

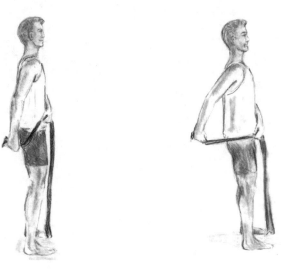

INSTRUCTION: Stand in neutral position. Wrap ends of resistive band around each hand. Place left hand next to right hip and extend straight right arm behind back. Repeat with opposite side.

HOLD: _____ second(s) **REPEAT:** _____ time(s) **FREQUENCY:** _____ x/day

SPECIAL PROTOCOLS/NOTES: <u>Do not round shoulders.</u>
_____
_____
_____

PATIENT NAME: _____ DATE: _____

THERAPIST NAME: _____

Standing Latisimus Dorsi Pull Down

PURPOSE: To strengthen shoulder muscles.

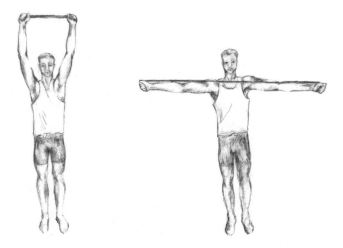

INSTRUCTION: Stand in neutral position. Grasp ends of resistive band with both hands. Raise both arms together overhead. Lower arms to shoulder height and pull band down in front of head.

HOLD: _____ second(s) **REPEAT:** _____ time(s) **FREQUENCY:** _____ x/day

SPECIAL PROTOCOLS/NOTES: Do not round shoulders. _____
_____
_____
_____

PATIENT NAME: _____ DATE: _____

THERAPIST NAME: _____

Standing Latisimus Dorsi Pull Down — Behind Head

PURPOSE: To strengthen shoulder muscles.

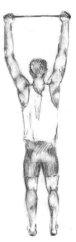 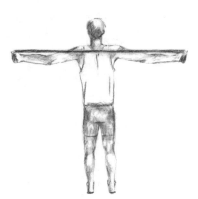

INSTRUCTION: Stand in neutral position. Grasp ends of resistive band with both hands. Raise both arms overhead. Lower arms to shoulder height and pull band down behind head.

HOLD: _____ second(s) **REPEAT:** _____ time(s) **FREQUENCY:** _____ x/day

SPECIAL PROTOCOLS/NOTES: Do not round shoulders. _____

_____

_____

_____

PATIENT NAME: _____   DATE: _____

THERAPIST NAME: _____

Standing Supraspinatus Exercise

PURPOSE: To strengthen arm and shoulder muscles.

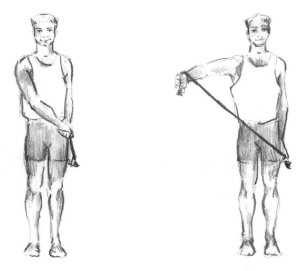

INSTRUCTION: Stand in neutral position. Wrap ends of resistive band around each hand. Place both hands on left hip. Rotate right thumb down. Raise right hand to shoulder height, keeping arm at a 45° angle to body. Repeat with opposite side.

HOLD: _____ second(s) **REPEAT:** _____ time(s) **FREQUENCY:** _____ x/day

SPECIAL PROTOCOLS/NOTES: _____
_____
_____
_____

PATIENT NAME: _____ DATE: _____
THERAPIST NAME: _____

Standing Shoulder Abduction to 90°

PURPOSE: To strengthen arm and shoulder muscles.

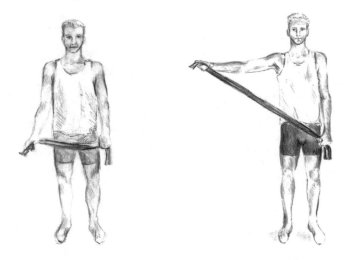

INSTRUCTION: Stand in neutral position. Wrap ends of resistive band around each hand. Move hand out away from body with thumb pointing toward ceiling. Raise right arm to 90°. Repeat with opposite side.

HOLD: _____ second(s) **REPEAT:** _____ time(s) **FREQUENCY:** _____ x/day

SPECIAL PROTOCOLS/NOTES: Do not round shoulders. _____

_____

_____

_____

PATIENT NAME: _____ DATE: _____

THERAPIST NAME: _____

Standing Shoulder Abduction

PURPOSE: To strengthen arm and shoulder muscles.

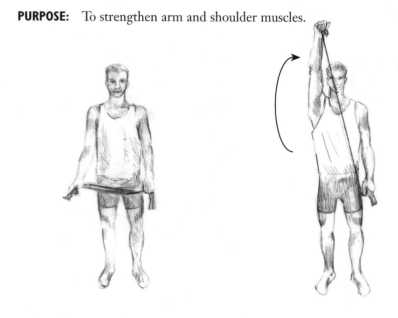

INSTRUCTION: Stand in neutral position. Wrap ends of resistive band around each hand. Move right hand out away from body with thumb pointing toward ceiling. Raise right arm overhead. Repeat with opposite side.

HOLD: _____ second(s) **REPEAT:** _____ time(s) **FREQUENCY:** _____ x/day

SPECIAL PROTOCOLS/NOTES: Do not round shoulders. _____

_____

_____

_____

PATIENT NAME: _____ DATE: _____

THERAPIST NAME: _____

Standing Horizontal Abduction

PURPOSE: To strengthen mid-back and shoulder muscles.

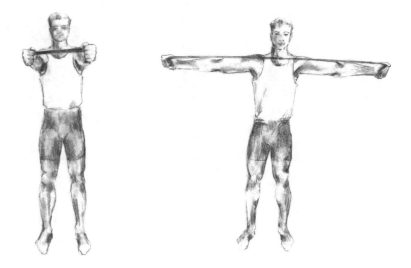

INSTRUCTION: Stand in neutral position. Grasp ends of resistive band with both hands. Raise both arms to shoulder height. Move arms out to sides of body.

HOLD: _____ second(s) **REPEAT:** _____ time(s) **FREQUENCY:** _____ x/day

SPECIAL PROTOCOLS/NOTES: Do not round shoulders.

_____

_____

_____

VARIATION: Follow directions as above, however, move each arm out to side of body one at a time.

PATIENT NAME: _____ DATE: _____

THERAPIST NAME: _____

Standing Lateral Raise

PURPOSE: To strengthen arm, mid-back, and shoulder muscles.

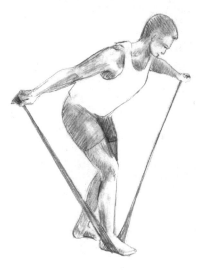

INSTRUCTION: Stand with right foot in front of the left foot. Wrap ends of resistive band around each hand. Loop band underneath right forefoot. Bend knees slightly and lean forward at waist. Straighten both arms and raise together up and away from sides of body. Repeat with opposite side.

HOLD: _____ second(s) **REPEAT:** _____ time(s) **FREQUENCY:** _____ x/day

SPECIAL PROTOCOLS/NOTES: Do not round back. Do not raise shoulders toward ear._____

_____

_____

PATIENT NAME: _____ DATE: _____

THERAPIST NAME: _____

Standing Shoulder Horizontal Adduction

PURPOSE: To strengthen chest and shoulder muscles.

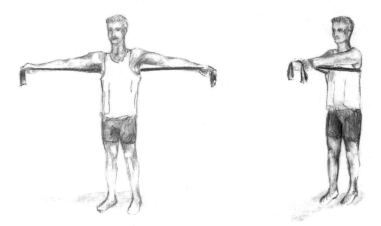

INSTRUCTION: Stand in neutral position. Wrap ends of resistive band around each hand. Loop band around back. Raise both arms out to sides at shoulder height. Move arms from sides of body to front of body.

HOLD: _____ second(s) **REPEAT:** _____ time(s) **FREQUENCY:** _____ x/day

SPECIAL PROTOCOLS/NOTES: Do not round shoulders. _____

_____

_____

_____

PATIENT NAME: _____   DATE: _____

THERAPIST NAME: _____

Standing Shoulder Horizontal Adduction Crossing Arms in Front of Body

PURPOSE: To strengthen chest and shoulder muscles.

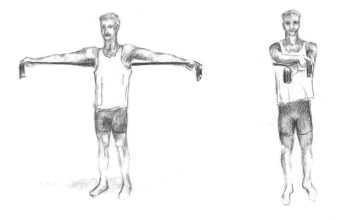

INSTRUCTION: Stand in neutral position. Wrap ends of resistive band around each hand. Loop band around back. Raise both arms out at sides to shoulder height. Move arms from sides of body to front of body. Cross arms in front of body.

HOLD: _____ second(s) **REPEAT:** _____ time(s) **FREQUENCY:** _____ x/day

SPECIAL PROTOCOLS/NOTES: Do not round shoulders.

_____
_____
_____

PATIENT NAME: _____   DATE: _____

THERAPIST NAME: _____

Standing Shoulder Internal Rotation

PURPOSE: To strengthen shoulder muscles.

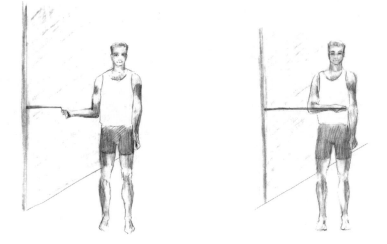

INSTRUCTION: Tie knot in one end of resistive band and shut knot in door at elbow height. Stand in neutral position with right side facing door. Wrap other end of band around right hand. Bend elbow and bring hand in toward abdomen. Repeat with opposite side.

HOLD: _____ second(s) **REPEAT:** _____ time(s) **FREQUENCY:** _____ x/day

SPECIAL PROTOCOLS/NOTES: Do not round shoulders. _____

_____

_____

_____

PATIENT NAME: _____ DATE: _____

THERAPIST NAME: _____

Standing Shoulder Internal Rotation with 90° of Shoulder Abduction

PURPOSE: To strengthen shoulder muscles.

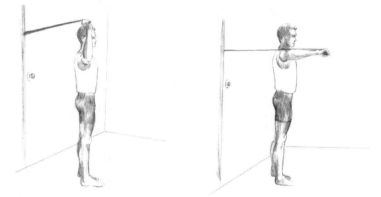

INSTRUCTION: Tie knot in one end of resistive band and shut knot in door at shoulder height. Stand in neutral position facing away from door. Wrap other end of band around right hand. Bend right elbow, and raise arm out away from body to form a 90° angle. Lower hand keeping elbow stationary. Repeat with opposite side.

HOLD: _____ second(s) **REPEAT:** _____ time(s) **FREQUENCY:** _____ x/day

SPECIAL PROTOCOLS/NOTES: Do not elevate shoulders.

_____
_____
_____

PATIENT NAME: _____ DATE: _____

THERAPIST NAME: _____

Standing Shoulder External Rotation

PURPOSE: To strengthen shoulder muscles.

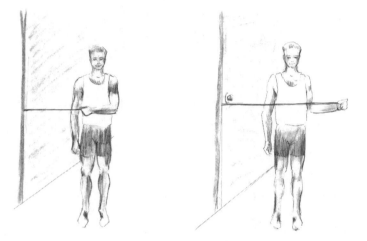

INSTRUCTION: Tie knot in one end of resistive band and shut knot in door at elbow height. Stand in neutral position with right side facing door. Wrap other end of band around left hand. Bend left elbow and move hand away from abdomen. Repeat with opposite side.

HOLD: _____ second(s) **REPEAT:** _____ time(s) **FREQUENCY:** _____ x/day

SPECIAL PROTOCOLS/NOTES: Do not slouch. _____

_____

_____

_____

PATIENT NAME: _____ DATE: _____

THERAPIST NAME: _____

Standing Shoulder External Rotation with 90° of Shoulder Abduction

PURPOSE: To strengthen shoulder muscles.

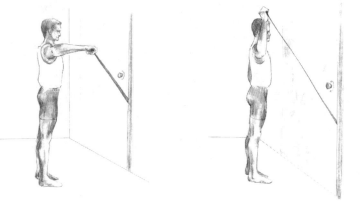

INSTRUCTION: Tie knot in one end of resistive band and shut in door at waist height. Stand in neutral position facing door. Wrap other end of band around right hand. Bend right elbow with palm down. Raise arm out away from body to form a 90° angle. Raise hand toward ceiling, keeping elbow stationary. Repeat with opposite side.

HOLD: _____ second(s) **REPEAT:** _____ time(s) **FREQUENCY:** _____ x/day

SPECIAL PROTOCOLS/NOTES: Do not elevate shoulders. _____

_____
_____
_____

PATIENT NAME: _____ DATE: _____

THERAPIST NAME: _____

Standing Bilateral Shoulder External Rotation

PURPOSE: To strengthen shoulder muscles.

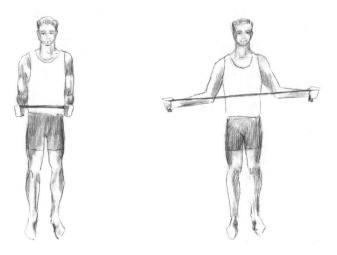

INSTRUCTION: Wrap ends of resistive band around each hand. Stand in neutral position. Bend elbows next to sides of body. Move both hands away from abdomen keeping elbows next to body. Return to starting position.

HOLD: _____ second(s) **REPEAT:** _____ time(s) **FREQUENCY:** _____ x/day

SPECIAL PROTOCOLS/NOTES: Do not slouch. _____
_____
_____
_____

PATIENT NAME: _____ DATE: _____

THERAPIST NAME: _____

Standing Shoulder Protraction

PURPOSE: To strengthen shoulder muscles.

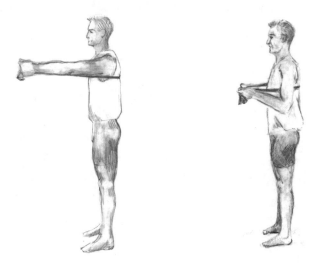

INSTRUCTION: Stand in neutral position. Grasp ends of resistive band with both hands. Loop band behind back. Bend elbows and push hands foward.

HOLD: _____ second(s) **REPEAT:** _____ time(s) **FREQUENCY:** _____ x/day

SPECIAL PROTOCOLS/NOTES: Do not round shoulders. _____

_____

_____

_____

VARIATION: Follow instructions as above, however push only one hand forward at a time.

PATIENT NAME: _____ DATE: _____

THERAPIST NAME: _____

Standing Shoulder Protraction
Crossing Arms
in Front of Body

PURPOSE: To strengthen shoulder muscles.

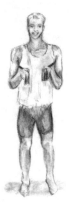 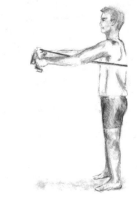

INSTRUCTION: Stand in neutral position. Grasp ends of resistive band with both hands. Loop band behind back. Bend elbows and push hands foward crossing hands in front of body. Alternate crossing right hand over left, and left hand over right.

HOLD: _____ second(s) **REPEAT:** _____ time(s) **FREQUENCY:** _____ x/day

SPECIAL PROTOCOLS/NOTES: <u>Do not round shoulders.</u>

_____

_____

_____

PATIENT NAME: _____ DATE: _____

THERAPIST NAME: _____

Standing Shoulder Protraction Crossing Arms and Raising Overhead

PURPOSE: To strengthen arm, chest, and shoulder muscles.

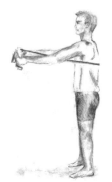 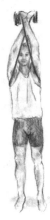

INSTRUCTION: Stand in neutral position. Wrap ends of resistive band around each hand. Loop band behind back. Bend elbows and push hands forward crossing hands in front of body. Raise both hands overhead. Alternate crossing right hand over left, and left hand over right.

HOLD: _____ second(s) **REPEAT:** _____ time(s) **FREQUENCY:** _____ x/day

SPECIAL PROTOCOLS/NOTES: Do not round shoulders. _____

_____

_____

_____

PATIENT NAME: _____   DATE: _____

THERAPIST NAME: _____

Standing Pectoralis Fly

PURPOSE: To strengthen chest and shoulder muscles.

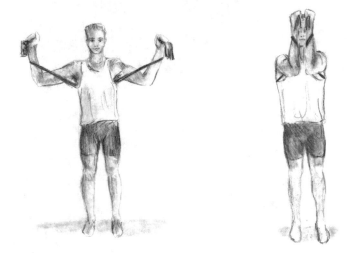

INSTRUCTION: Stand in neutral position. Grasp ends of resistive band with hands and forearms. Loop band around back and under arms. Bend elbows and raise both arms to shoulder height. Move elbows from sides of body to front of body.

HOLD: _____ second(s) **REPEAT:** _____ time(s) **FREQUENCY:** _____ x/day

SPECIAL PROTOCOLS/NOTES: Do not round shoulders. _____
_____
_____
_____

PATIENT NAME: _____ DATE: _____

THERAPIST NAME: _____

Standing Push-Up

PURPOSE: To strengthen arm, chest, forearm, and shoulder muscles.

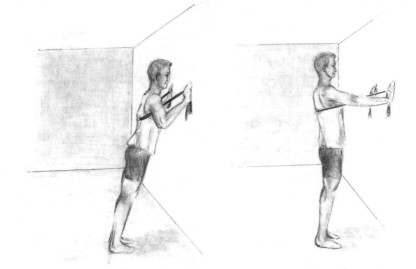

INSTRUCTION:-.Stand facing wall in neutral position with feet shoulder-width apart and several feet from wall. Grasp ends of resistive band with both hands. Loop band behind back. Lean forward with elbows bent and place hands on wall. Do a push-up.

HOLD: _____ second(s) **REPEAT:** _____ time(s) **FREQUENCY:** _____ x/day

SPECIAL PROTOCOLS/NOTES: Do not arch back or slouch. _____

_____

_____

_____

PATIENT NAME: _____   DATE: _____

THERAPIST NAME: _____

Standing Shoulder Blade Squeeze

PURPOSE: To strengthen mid-back and shoulder muscles.

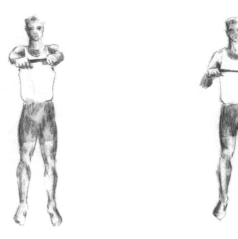

INSTRUCTION: Grasp resistive band with both hands. Stand in neutral position. Raise both arms to shoulder height. Bend elbows and pull backward, while squeezing shoulder blades together.

HOLD: _____ second(s) **REPEAT:** _____ time(s) **FREQUENCY:** _____ x/day

SPECIAL PROTOCOLS/NOTES: Do not slouch. _____

_____

_____

_____

PATIENT NAME: _____ DATE: _____

THERAPIST NAME: _____

Standing Unilateral Shoulder Rowing

PURPOSE: To strengthen arm, shoulder, and mid-back muscles.

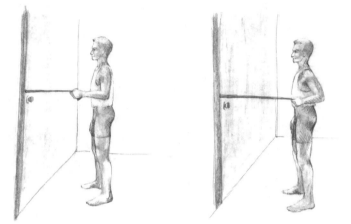

INSTRUCTION: Tie knot in one end of resistive band and shut knot in door at elbow height. Stand in neutral position, facing door. Wrap other end of band around left hand. Bend left elbow and pull backward. Repeat with opposite side.

HOLD: _____ second(s) **REPEAT:** _____ time(s) **FREQUENCY:** _____ x/day

SPECIAL PROTOCOLS/NOTES: <u>Do not slouch.</u>

_____
_____
_____

PATIENT NAME: _____   DATE: _____

THERAPIST NAME: _____

Standing Unilateral Shoulder Rowing with Trunk Flexion

PURPOSE: To strengthen arm, shoulder, and mid-back muscles.

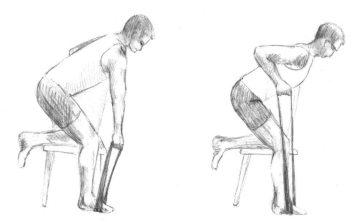

INSTRUCTION: Stand in neutral position with left knee on chair. Grasp the ends of resistive band with right hand. Loop resistive around right foot. Bend forward at waist without rounding back. Bend elbows and pull backward. Repeat with opposite side.

HOLD: _____ second(s) **REPEAT:** _____ time(s) **FREQUENCY:** _____ x/day

SPECIAL PROTOCOLS/NOTES: Do not slouch._____

_____

_____

_____

PATIENT NAME: _____ DATE: _____

THERAPIST NAME: _____

Standing Bilateral Shoulder Rowing

PURPOSE: To strengthen arm, shoulder, and mid-back muscles.

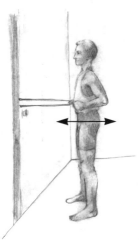

INSTRUCTION: Tie knot in middle of resistive band and shut knot in door at elbow height. Stand in neutral position, facing door. Wrap ends of band around each hand. Bend elbows and pull backward.

HOLD: _____ second(s) **REPEAT:** _____ time(s) **FREQUENCY:** _____ x/day

SPECIAL PROTOCOLS/NOTES: Do not slouch. _____
_____
_____
_____

PATIENT NAME: _____ DATE: _____

THERAPIST NAME: _____

Standing Bow Exercise

PURPOSE: To strengthen arm and shoulder muscles.

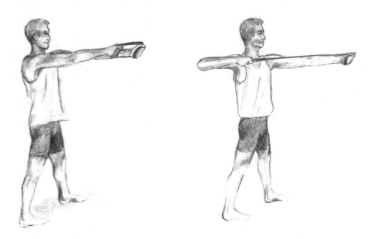

INSTRUCTION: Stand in neutral position with left foot in front of right foot. Grasp ends of resistive band with each hand. Raise both arms to shoulder height. Rotate left thumb toward ceiling. Bend right elbow and pull back. Repeat with opposite side.

HOLD: _____ second(s) **REPEAT:** _____ time(s) **FREQUENCY:** _____ x/day

SPECIAL PROTOCOLS/NOTES: _____

_____

_____

_____

PATIENT NAME: _____ DATE: _____

THERAPIST NAME: _____

Standing Lawnmower Pull

PURPOSE: To strengthen mid-back and arm muscles.

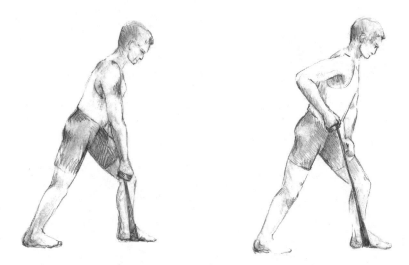

INSTRUCTION: Stand with left foot in front of right foot. Wrap one end of resistive band around right hand. Step on other end of band with left forefoot. Lean forward at waist. Bend right elbow and pull backward. Repeat with opposite side.

HOLD: _____ second(s) **REPEAT:** _____ time(s) **FREQUENCY:** _____ x/day

SPECIAL PROTOCOLS/NOTES: Do not round back. Do not raise shoulder toward ear. _____
_____
_____

PATIENT NAME: _____ DATE: _____

THERAPIST NAME: _____

Standing Shoulder PNF Diagonal One — Flexion

PURPOSE: To strengthen shoulder muscles.

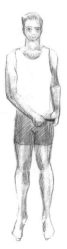 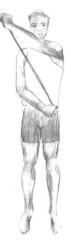

INSTRUCTION: Stand in neutral position. Grasp ends of resistive band with both hands. Place right hand on left hip. Raise left hand up and over right shoulder. Repeat with opposite side.

HOLD: _____ second(s) **REPEAT:** _____ time(s) **FREQUENCY:** _____ x/day

SPECIAL PROTOCOLS/NOTES: Do not round shoulders. _____

_____

_____

_____

PATIENT NAME: _____ DATE: _____

THERAPIST NAME: _____

Standing Shoulder Diagonal Two — Flexion

PURPOSE: To strengthen shoulder muscles.

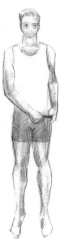 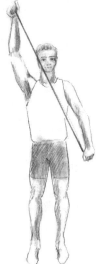

INSTRUCTION: Stand in neutral position. Grasp ends of resistive band with both hands. Lower left hand down by left hip. Place right hand by left hip. Raise right hand overhead. Repeat with opposite side.

HOLD: _____ second(s) **REPEAT:** _____ time(s) **FREQUENCY:** _____ x/day

SPECIAL PROTOCOLS/NOTES: Do not round shoulders. _____

_____

_____

_____

PATIENT NAME: _____ DATE: _____

THERAPIST NAME: _____

Standing Shoulder PNF Diagonal One — Extension

PURPOSE: To strengthen shoulder muscles.

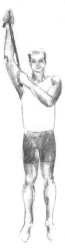 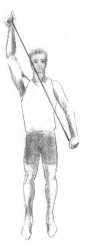

INSTRUCTION: Stand in neutral position. Grasp ends of resistive band with both hands. Raise right arm overhead and place left hand on right shoulder with elbow bent. Pull left hand down to left side of hip. Repeat with opposite side.

HOLD: _____ second(s) **REPEAT:** _____ time(s) **FREQUENCY:** _____ x/day

SPECIAL PROTOCOLS/NOTES: Do not round shoulders. _____

_____

_____

_____

PATIENT NAME: _____ DATE: _____

THERAPIST NAME: _____

Standing Shoulder PNF Diagonal Two — Extension

PURPOSE: To strengthen shoulder muscles.

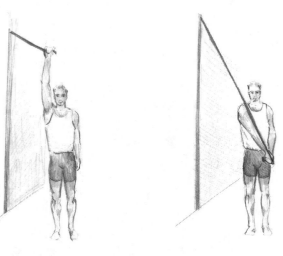

INSTRUCTION: Stand in neutral position. Grasp ends of resistive band with both hands. Raise right arm overhead and place left hand on right shoulder with elbow bent. Pull left hand down to left side of hip. Repeat with opposite side.

HOLD: _____ second(s) **REPEAT:** _____ time(s) **FREQUENCY:** _____ x/day

SPECIAL PROTOCOLS/NOTES: Do not round shoulders. _____
_____
_____
_____

PATIENT NAME: _____ DATE: _____
THERAPIST NAME: _____

Standing Trunk Side Bends

PURPOSE: To strengthen trunk muscles.

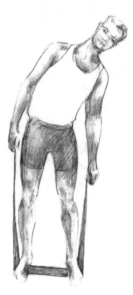

INSTRUCTION: Stand in neutral position. Grasp ends of resistive band with both hands. Loop band under both feet, standing on band. Side bend to one side. Repeat in opposite direction.

HOLD: _____ second(s) **REPEAT:** _____ time(s) **FREQUENCY:** _____ x/day

SPECIAL PROTOCOLS/NOTES: Do not round back. _____
_____
_____
_____

PATIENT NAME: _____ DATE: _____
THERAPIST NAME: _____

Standing Trunk Rotation — Diagonal One

PURPOSE: To strengthen abdominal, back, and trunk muscles.

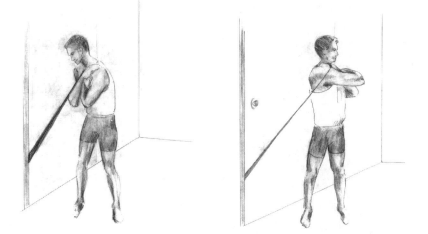

INSTRUCTION: Tie knot in one end of resistive band and shut knot in door at knee height. Wrap other end of band around left hand. Stand in neutral position with right hip toward door. Bend at waist and rotate trunk toward right hip. Straighten at waist and rotate trunk and head over left shoulder. Repeat with opposite side.

HOLD: _____ second(s) **REPEAT:** _____ time(s) **FREQUENCY:** _____ x/day

SPECIAL PROTOCOLS/NOTES: Do not rotate hips with upper body. Keep hips facing forward and arms close to body.

_____

_____

PATIENT NAME: _____ DATE: _____

THERAPIST NAME: _____

Standing Trunk Rotation — Diagonal Two

PURPOSE: To strengthen abdominal, back, and trunk muscles.

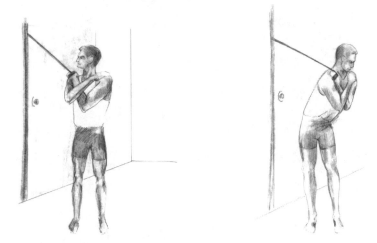

INSTRUCTION: Tie knot in one end of resistive band and shut knot in door at highest point. Wrap other end of band around left hand. Stand in neutral position with right hip toward door. Bend at waist and rotate trunk down toward left hip. Repeat with opposite side.

HOLD: _____ second(s) **REPEAT:** _____ time(s) **FREQUENCY:** _____ x/day

SPECIAL PROTOCOLS/NOTES: Do not rotate hips with upper body. Keep hips facing forward and arms close to body.

_____

_____

PATIENT NAME: _____ DATE: _____

THERAPIST NAME: _____

Standing Unilateral Squat

PURPOSE: To strengthen buttock, leg, and thigh muscles.

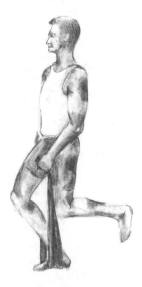

INSTRUCTION: Stand in neutral position. Grasp ends of resistive band with both hands. Loop band under right foot and stand on band. Lift left foot off floor with knee bent. Bend right knee slightly. Repeat with opposite side.

HOLD: _____ second(s) **REPEAT:** _____ time(s) **FREQUENCY:** _____ x/day

SPECIAL PROTOCOLS/NOTES: Do not round back. _____

_____

_____

_____

VARIATION: Follow directions as above. Bend both knees into a full squat position.

PATIENT NAME: _____   DATE: _____

THERAPIST NAME: _____

Standing Squat

PURPOSE: To strengthen buttock, leg, and thigh muscles.

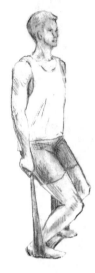

INSTRUCTION: Stand in neutral position. Grasp ends of resistive band with both hands. Loop band under both feet, standing on band and keeping feet shoulder-width apart. Bend both knees slightly.

HOLD: _____ second(s) **REPEAT:** _____ time(s) **FREQUENCY:** _____ x/day

SPECIAL PROTOCOLS/NOTES: Do not round back.

_____

_____

_____

VARIATION: Follow directions as above. Bend both knees into a full squat position.

PATIENT NAME: _____   DATE: _____

THERAPIST NAME: _____

Standing Squat with Ball

PURPOSE: To strengthen buttock, leg, and thigh muscles.

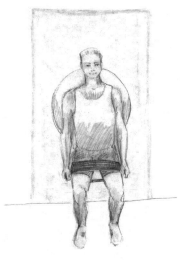

INSTRUCTION: Stand near a wall, facing away from it in neutral position with feet shoulder-width apart. Loop resistive band around knees. Place ball against wall behind small curve of back. Bend both knees slightly.

HOLD: _____ second(s) **REPEAT:** _____ time(s) **FREQUENCY:** _____ x/day

SPECIAL PROTOCOLS/NOTES: Do not round back.

_____

_____

_____

VARIATION: Follow directions as above. Bend both knees into a full squat position.

PATIENT NAME: _____ DATE: _____

THERAPIST NAME: _____

Standing Squat with Two Balls

PURPOSE: To strengthen buttock, leg, and thigh muscles.

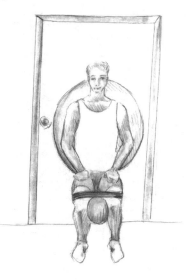

INSTRUCTION: Stand near a wall in neutral position with feet shoulder-width apart. Loop resistive band around knees and place small ball between knees. Place large ball against wall behind small curve of back. Bend both knees slightly.

HOLD: _____ second(s) **REPEAT:** _____ time(s) **FREQUENCY:** _____ x/day

SPECIAL PROTOCOLS/NOTES: Do not round back. _____

_____

_____

_____

VARIATION: Follow directions as above. Bend both knees into a full squat position.

PATIENT NAME: _____ DATE: _____

THERAPIST NAME: _____

Standing Plié

PURPOSE: To strengthen buttock, leg, and thigh muscles.

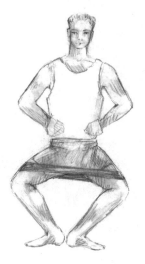

INSTRUCTION: Stand in neutral position. Loop resistive band around both lower thighs. Place heels together and rotate toes away from each other. Bend knees, keeping knees in line with feet.

HOLD: _____ second(s) **REPEAT:** _____ time(s) **FREQUENCY:** _____ x/day

SPECIAL PROTOCOLS/NOTES: Do not round back. _____

_____

_____

_____

PATIENT NAME: _____	DATE: _____
THERAPIST NAME: _____	

Standing Hip Abduction/Adduction

PURPOSE: To strengthen hip muscles.

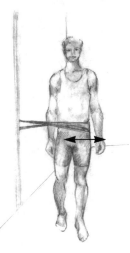

INSTRUCTION: Tie both ends of resistive band together and shut knot in door at hip height. Stand in neutral position with right side of body toward door. Loop band around hips. Stand with most of body weight on left foot, taking weight off right foot by placing only toes on floor. Gently oscillate left hip side to side. Repeat with opposite side.

HOLD: _____ second(s) **REPEAT:** _____ time(s) **FREQUENCY:** _____ x/day

SPECIAL PROTOCOLS/NOTES: Do not slouch. _____

_____

_____

_____

PATIENT NAME: _____ DATE: _____

THERAPIST NAME: _____

Standing Hip Flexion
with Band Around Ankle

PURPOSE: To strengthen hip, front of thigh, and leg muscles.

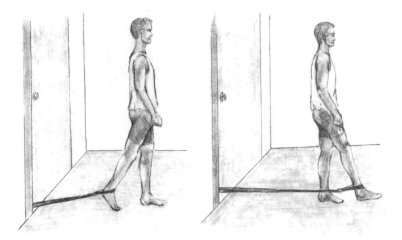

INSTRUCTION: Tie knot in one end of resistive band and shut knot in door. With other end of band, make a loop and wrap around right ankle. Stand with feet shoulder-width apart, facing away from door. Raise right foot toward ceiling. Return to starting position. Repeat with opposite side.

HOLD: _____ second(s) **REPEAT:** _____ time(s) **FREQUENCY:** _____ x/day

SPECIAL PROTOCOLS/NOTES: <u>Do not round back while raising leg.</u>

_____

_____

_____

PATIENT NAME: _____ DATE: _____

THERAPIST NAME: _____

Standing Hip Flexion with Band Around Thigh

PURPOSE: To strengthen hip and front of thigh muscles.

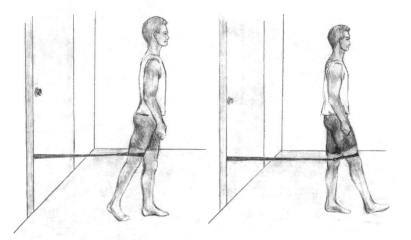

INSTRUCTION: Tie knot in one end of resistive band and shut knot in door. With other end of band, make a loop and wrap around right thigh. Stand with feet shoulder-width apart, facing away from door. Raise right foot toward ceiling. Return to starting position. Repeat with opposite side.

HOLD: _____ second(s) **REPEAT:** _____ time(s) **FREQUENCY:** _____ x/day

SPECIAL PROTOCOLS/NOTES: <u>Do not round back while raising leg.</u>

_____

_____

_____

PATIENT NAME: _____ DATE: _____

THERAPIST NAME: _____

Standing Hip Extension with Band Around Ankle

PURPOSE: To strengthen hip, back of thigh, and leg muscles.

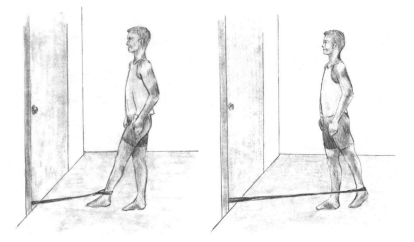

INSTRUCTION: Tie knot in one end of resistive band and shut knot in door. With other end of band, make a loop and wrap around left ankle. Stand with feet shoulder-width apart, facing door. Extend left leg behind back. Raise left heel toward ceiling. Return to starting position. Repeat with opposite side.

HOLD: _____ second(s) **REPEAT:** _____ time(s) **FREQUENCY:** _____ x/day

SPECIAL PROTOCOLS/NOTES: Do not arch back. Keep leg straight.

_____

_____

_____

PATIENT NAME: _____   DATE: _____

THERAPIST NAME: _____

Standing Hip Extension with Band Around Thigh

PURPOSE: To strengthen hip, back of thigh, and leg muscles.

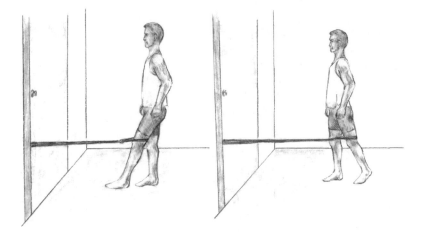

INSTRUCTION: Tie knot in one end of resistive band and shut knot in door. With other end of band, make a loop and wrap around left thigh. Stand with feet shoulder-width apart, facing door. Extend left leg behind back. Raise left heel toward ceiling. Return to starting position. Repeat with opposite side.

HOLD: _____ second(s) **REPEAT:** _____ time(s) **FREQUENCY:** _____ x/day

SPECIAL PROTOCOLS/NOTES: Do not arch back. Keep leg straight.

_____
_____
_____

PATIENT NAME: _____ DATE: _____

THERAPIST NAME: _____

Standing Hip Abduction
with Band Around Ankle

PURPOSE: To strengthen hip, outer thigh, and leg muscles.

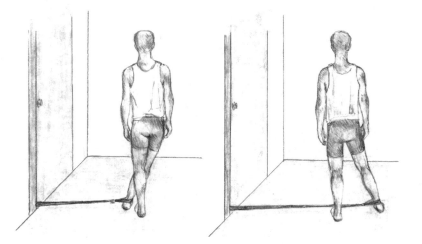

INSTRUCTION: Tie knot in one end of resistive band and shut knot in door. With other end of band, make a loop and wrap around right ankle. Stand with right outer thigh away from door. Raise right ankle toward ceiling. Return to starting position. Repeat with opposite side.

HOLD: _____ second(s) **REPEAT:** _____ time(s) **FREQUENCY:** _____ x/day

SPECIAL PROTOCOLS/NOTES: Keep leg straight and aligned with opposite leg. _____
_____
_____

PATIENT NAME: _____ DATE: _____

THERAPIST NAME: _____

Standing Hip Abduction with Band Around Thigh

PURPOSE: To strengthen hip, outer thigh, and leg muscles.

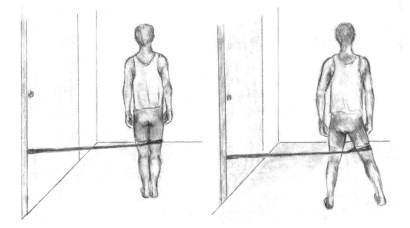

INSTRUCTION: Tie knot in one end of resistive band and shut knot in door. With other end of band, make a loop and wrap around right thigh. Stand with right outer thigh away from door. Raise right ankle toward ceiling. Return to starting position. Repeat with opposite side.

HOLD: _____ second(s) **REPEAT:** _____ time(s) **FREQUENCY:** _____ x/day

SPECIAL PROTOCOLS/NOTES: Keep leg straight and aligned with opposite leg.
_____
_____

PATIENT NAME: _____ DATE: _____

THERAPIST NAME: _____

Standing Hip Adduction with Band Around Ankle

PURPOSE: To strengthen hip and inner thigh muscles.

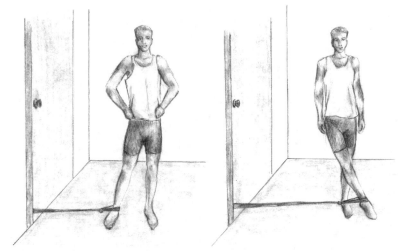

INSTRUCTION: Tie knot in one end of resistive band and shut knot in door. With other end of band, make a loop and wrap around right ankle. Stand with right outer thigh toward door. Cross right leg over left. Return to starting position. Repeat with opposite side.

HOLD: _____ second(s) **REPEAT:** _____ time(s) **FREQUENCY:** _____ x/day

SPECIAL PROTOCOLS/NOTES: Keep leg straight. Do not rotate hips.

_____

_____

_____

PATIENT NAME: _____ DATE: _____

THERAPIST NAME: _____

Standing Hip Adduction with Band Around Thigh

PURPOSE: To strengthen hip and inner thigh muscles.

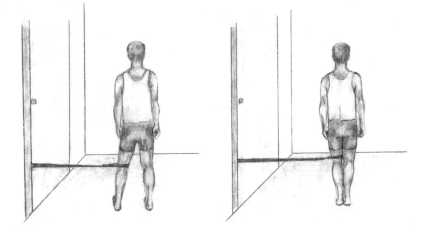

INSTRUCTION: Tie knot in one end of resistive band and shut knot in door. With other end of band, make a loop and wrap around right thigh. Stand with right outer thigh toward door. Cross right leg over left. Return to starting position. Repeat with opposite side.

HOLD: _____ second(s) **REPEAT:** _____ time(s) **FREQUENCY:** _____ x/day

SPECIAL PROTOCOLS/NOTES: Keep leg straight. Do not rotate hips. _____

_____

_____

_____

PATIENT NAME: _____ DATE: _____

THERAPIST NAME: _____

Standing Knee Raise

PURPOSE: To strengthen hip and front of thigh muscles.

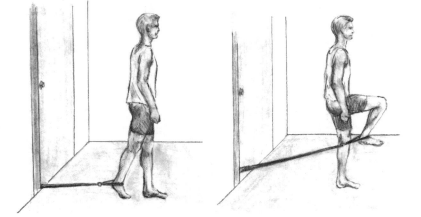

INSTRUCTION: Tie knot in one end of resistive band and shut knot in door. With other end of band, make a loop and wrap around right ankle. Stand facing away from door. Bend right knee and raise toward ceiling. Return to starting position. Repeat with opposite side.

HOLD: _____ second(s) **REPEAT:** _____ time(s) **FREQUENCY:** _____ x/day

SPECIAL PROTOCOLS/NOTES: Do not round back while raising leg.

_____

_____

_____

PATIENT NAME: _____   DATE: _____

THERAPIST NAME: _____

Standing Knee Flexion

PURPOSE: To strengthen back of thigh muscles.

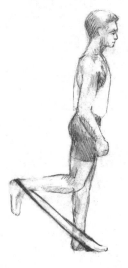

INSTRUCTION: Tie ends of resistive band together. Loop band around right ankle and left forefoot. Stand in neutral position. Bend right knee toward buttocks. Repeat with opposite side.

HOLD: _____ second(s) **REPEAT:** _____ time(s) **FREQUENCY:** _____ x/day

SPECIAL PROTOCOLS/NOTES: Do not lean forward or arch back. _____

_____

_____

_____

PATIENT NAME: _____ DATE: _____

THERAPIST NAME: _____

Standing Knee Flexion with Band Above Knee

PURPOSE: To strengthen knee and thigh muscles.

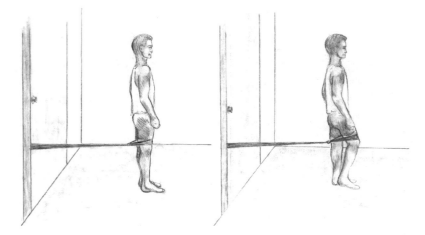

INSTRUCTION: Tie knot in one end of resistive band and shut knot in door. With other end of band, make a loop and wrap around right leg above knee. Stand with feet shoulder-width apart, facing away from door. Bend right knee. Slowly return knee to starting position. Repeat with opposite side.

HOLD: _____ second(s) **REPEAT:** _____ time(s) **FREQUENCY:** _____ x/day

SPECIAL PROTOCOLS/NOTES: Do not let band snap leg back. _____

_____

_____

_____

PATIENT NAME: _____ DATE: _____

THERAPIST NAME: _____

Standing Knee Flexion with Band Above and Below Knee

PURPOSE: To strengthen knee and thigh muscles.

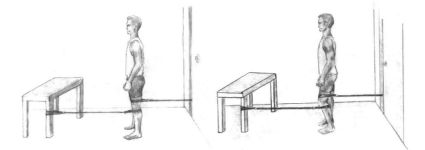

INSTRUCTION: Tie knot in one end of resistive band and shut knot in door. With other end of band, make a loop and wrap around right leg above knee. Loop second band around table leg, in opposite direction, and below right knee. Stand with feet shoulder-width apart, facing away from door. Bend right knee. Slowly return knee to starting position. Repeat with opposite side.

HOLD: _____ second(s) **REPEAT:** _____ time(s) **FREQUENCY:** _____ x/day

SPECIAL PROTOCOLS/NOTES: Do not let bands snap leg forward or backward.

PATIENT NAME: _____ DATE: _____

THERAPIST NAME: _____

Standing Knee Extension

PURPOSE: To strengthen knee and front thigh muscles.

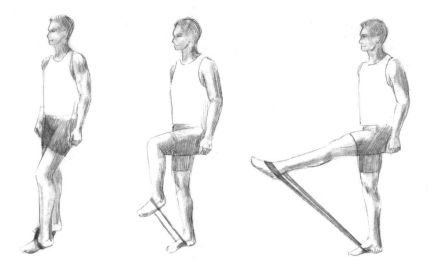

INSTRUCTION: Tie ends of resistive band together. Loop band around both forefeet. Stand in neutral position. Raise right knee and straighten. Repeat with opposite side.

HOLD: _____ second(s) **REPEAT:** _____ time(s) **FREQUENCY:** _____ x/day

SPECIAL PROTOCOLS/NOTES: Do not lean forward or arch back.

_____

_____

_____

PATIENT NAME: _____ DATE: _____

THERAPIST NAME: _____

111

Standing Knee Extension with Band Above Knee

PURPOSE: To strengthen knee and thigh muscles.

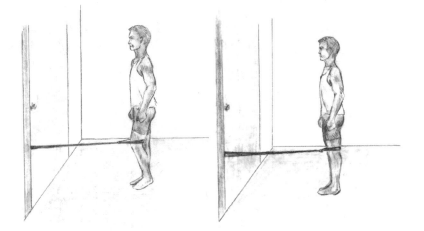

INSTRUCTION: Tie knot in one end of resistive band and shut knot in door. With other end of band, make a loop and wrap around left leg above knee. Stand with feet shoulder-width apart, facing door. Bend left knee. Slowly return knee to starting position. Repeat with opposite side.

HOLD: _____ second(s) **REPEAT:** _____ time(s) **FREQUENCY:** _____ x/day

SPECIAL PROTOCOLS/NOTES: Do not let band snap leg forward. _____

_____

_____

_____

PATIENT NAME: _____ DATE: _____

THERAPIST NAME: _____

Standing Knee Extension with Band Above and Below Knee

PURPOSE: To strengthen knee and thigh muscles.

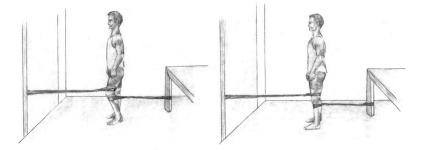

INSTRUCTION: Tie knot in one end of resistive band and shut knot in door. With other end of band, make a loop and wrap around left leg above knee. Loop second band around table leg, in opposite direction, and also below knee. Stand with feet shoulder-width apart, facing door. Bend knee, then slowly straighten. Repeat with opposite side.

HOLD: _____ second(s) **REPEAT:** _____ time(s) **FREQUENCY:** _____ x/day

SPECIAL PROTOCOLS/NOTES: Do not let band snap leg forward or
backward.
_____
_____
_____

PATIENT NAME: _____   DATE: _____

THERAPIST NAME: _____

Standing Heel Raises

PURPOSE: To strengthen calf muscles.

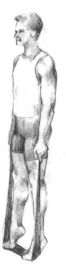

INSTRUCTION: Grasp ends of resistive band with both hands. Loop band under balls of both feet. Stand in neutral position. Raise heels off floor.

HOLD: _____ second(s) **REPEAT:** _____ time(s) **FREQUENCY:** _____ x/day

SPECIAL PROTOCOLS/NOTES: Do not lean forward or arch back.

_____

_____

_____

PATIENT NAME: _____ DATE: _____

THERAPIST NAME: _____

CHAPTER FOUR

Sitting Exercises

CHAPTER FOUR

LONG SITTING EXERCISES

Sitting Neutral Position

PURPOSE: To strengthen muscles in an optimal position to avoid injury.

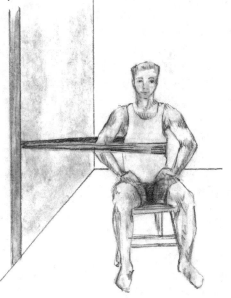

INSTRUCTION: Sit with feet shoulder-width apart and pointing forward. Align knees over feet. Maintain natural curve in back.

HOLD: _____ second(s) **REPEAT:** _____ time(s) **FREQUENCY:** _____ x/day

SPECIAL PROTOCOLS/NOTES: Do not arch back or slouch. _____
_____
_____
_____

PATIENT NAME: _____ DATE: _____
THERAPIST NAME: _____

Sitting Wrist Flexion

PURPOSE: To strengthen wrist muscles.

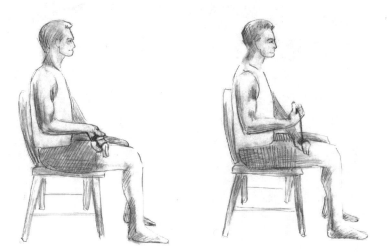

INSTRUCTION: Sit in neutral position. Wrap ends of resistive band around each hand. Bend right elbow with palm up. Bend right wrist and raise palm toward shoulder. Repeat with opposite side.

HOLD: _____ second(s) **REPEAT:** _____ time(s) **FREQUENCY:** _____ x/day

SPECIAL PROTOCOLS/NOTES: Do not lift forearm. _____
_____
_____
_____

PATIENT NAME: _____ DATE: _____

THERAPIST NAME: _____

Sitting Wrist Extension

PURPOSE: To strengthen wrist muscles.

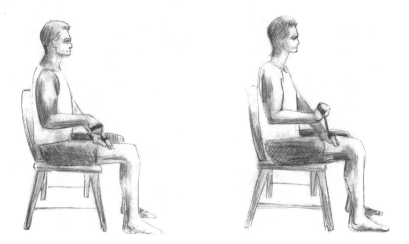

INSTRUCTION: Sit in neutral position. Wrap ends of resistive band around each hand. Bend right elbow with palm down. Bend right wrist and raise hand toward ceiling. Repeat with opposite side.

HOLD: _____ second(s) **REPEAT:** _____ time(s) **FREQUENCY:** _____ x/day

SPECIAL PROTOCOLS/NOTES: Do not lift forearm. _____

_____

_____

_____

PATIENT NAME: _____ DATE: _____

THERAPIST NAME: _____

Sitting Wrist Radial Deviation in Neutral

PURPOSE: To strengthen wrist muscles.

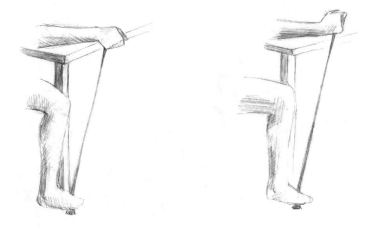

INSTRUCTION: Sit in neutral position. Place one end of resistive band under right foot and grasp other end of band with right hand. Bend right elbow, with thumb up, and place on table. Lower hand off table toward floor. Raise hand toward ceiling. Repeat with opposite side.

HOLD: _____ second(s) **REPEAT:** _____ time(s) **FREQUENCY:** _____ x/day

SPECIAL PROTOCOLS/NOTES: Do not lift forearm. Keep wrist in neutral position.

_____

_____

PATIENT NAME: _____ DATE: _____

THERAPIST NAME: _____

Sitting Wrist Ulnar Deviation in Neutral

PURPOSE: To strengthen wrist muscles.

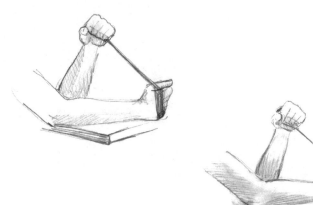

INSTRUCTION: Sit in neutral position. Wrap ends of resistive band around each hand. Bend elbows with thumbs up, and place on table. Place right forearm on table. Raise right hand toward ceiling, then lower hand off table toward floor. Repeat with opposite side.

HOLD: _____ second(s) **REPEAT:** _____ time(s) **FREQUENCY:** _____ x/day

SPECIAL PROTOCOLS/NOTES: Do not move forearm. _____
_____
_____
_____

PATIENT NAME: _____ DATE: _____
THERAPIST NAME: _____

Sitting Wrist Pronation

PURPOSE: To strengthen wrist muscles.

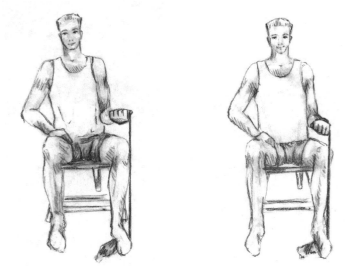

INSTRUCTION: Sit in neutral position with left foot on one end of resistive band. Bend left elbow with palm up. Wrap other end of band over top and around left hand. Rotate palm down. Repeat with opposite side.

HOLD: _____ second(s) **REPEAT:** _____ time(s) **FREQUENCY:** _____ x/day

SPECIAL PROTOCOLS/NOTES: Do not bend wrists. _____

_____

_____

_____

PATIENT NAME: _____ DATE: _____

THERAPIST NAME: _____

Sitting Wrist Supination

PURPOSE: To strengthen wrist muscles.

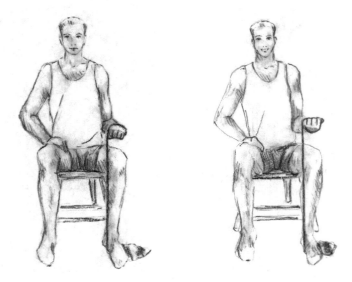

INSTRUCTION: Sit in neutral position with left foot on one end of resistive band. Bend left elbow with palm down. Wrap other end of band over top of left hand. Rotate palm up. Repeat with opposite side.

HOLD: _____ second(s) **REPEAT:** _____ time(s) **FREQUENCY:** _____ x/day

SPECIAL PROTOCOLS/NOTES: Do not lift forearm. _____

_____

_____

_____

PATIENT NAME: _____ DATE: _____

THERAPIST NAME: _____

Sitting Elbow Flexion

PURPOSE: To strengthen front of arm muscles.

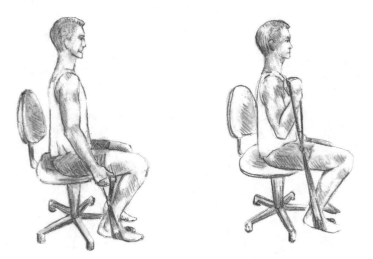

INSTRUCTION: Sit in neutral position. Loop resistive band around right hand and place other end of band under right foot. Bend right elbow with palm up. Raise hand toward shoulder. Repeat with opposite side.

HOLD: _____ second(s) **REPEAT:** _____ time(s) **FREQUENCY:** _____ x/day

SPECIAL PROTOCOLS/NOTES: _____

_____

_____

_____

PATIENT NAME: _____ DATE: _____

THERAPIST NAME: _____

Sitting Elbow Flexion with Palm Down

PURPOSE: To strengthen front of arm muscles.

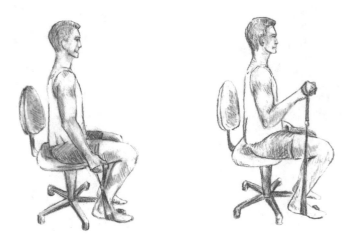

INSTRUCTION: Sit in neutral position. Loop resistive band around right hand and place other end of band under right foot. Bend right elbow with palm down. Raise hand toward shoulder. Repeat with opposite side.

HOLD: _____ second(s) **REPEAT:** _____ time(s) **FREQUENCY:** _____ x/day

SPECIAL PROTOCOLS/NOTES: _____
_____
_____
_____

PATIENT NAME: _____ DATE: _____

THERAPIST NAME: _____

Sitting Elbow Extension

PURPOSE: To strengthen back of arm muscles.

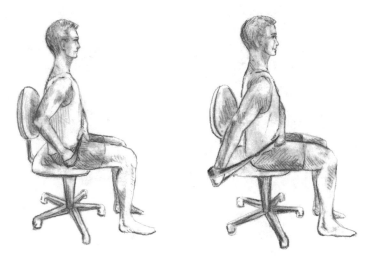

INSTRUCTION: Sit in neutral position. Wrap ends of resistive band around each hand. Place left hand on right hip. Extend right arm behind back. Repeat with opposite side.

HOLD: _____ second(s) **REPEAT:** _____ time(s) **FREQUENCY:** _____ x/day

SPECIAL PROTOCOLS/NOTES: Do not slouch. _____
_____
_____
_____

PATIENT NAME: _____ DATE: _____

THERAPIST NAME: _____

Sitting Shoulder Flexion

PURPOSE: To strengthen arm and shoulder muscles.

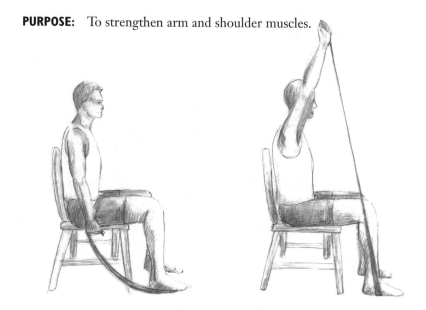

INSTRUCTION: Sit in neutral position. Grasp one end of resistive band with right hand and place other end of band under right foot. Begin with right arm straight down next to side of body. Raise arm overhead. Repeat with opposite side.

HOLD: _____ second(s) **REPEAT:** _____ time(s) **FREQUENCY:** _____ x/day

SPECIAL PROTOCOLS/NOTES: Do not slouch. _____

_____

_____

_____

PATIENT NAME: _____ DATE: _____

THERAPIST NAME: _____

Sitting Shoulder Extension

PURPOSE: To strengthen arm and shoulder muscles.

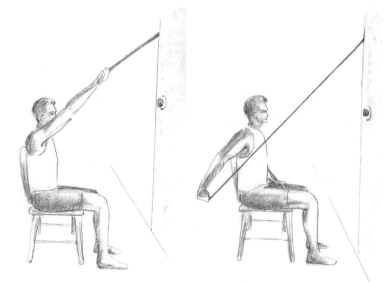

INSTRUCTION: Tie knot in one end of resistive band and shut knot in door. Sit in neutral position. Wrap other end of band around right hand. Raise right arm overhead. Pull band straight down behind back. Repeat with opposite side.

HOLD: _____ second(s) **REPEAT:** _____ time(s) **FREQUENCY:** _____ x/day

SPECIAL PROTOCOLS/NOTES: Do not slouch. _____

_____

_____

_____

PATIENT NAME: _____   DATE: _____

THERAPIST NAME: _____

Sitting Shoulder Abduction

PURPOSE: To strengthen shoulder muscles.

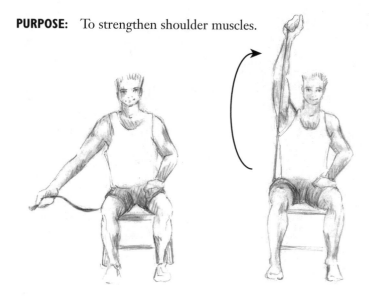

INSTRUCTION: Sit in neutral position. Sit on one end of resistive band and grasp other end of band with right hand. Raise right arm from side of body to overhead. Repeat with opposite side.

HOLD: _____ second(s) **REPEAT:** _____ time(s) **FREQUENCY:** _____ x/day

SPECIAL PROTOCOLS/NOTES: Do not slouch. _____

_____

_____

_____

PATIENT NAME: _____ DATE: _____

THERAPIST NAME: _____

Sitting Shoulder Adduction

PURPOSE: To strengthen shoulder muscles.

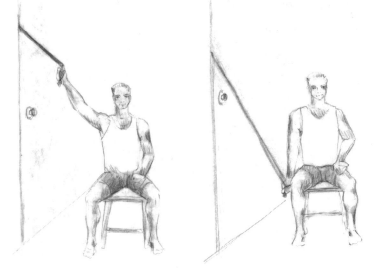

INSTRUCTION: Tie knot in one end of resistive band and shut knot in door. Sit in neutral position with right side of body toward door. Grasp other end of band with right hand. Raise right arm overhead. Pull band down to right side of body. Repeat with opposite side.

HOLD: _____ second(s) **REPEAT:** _____ time(s) **FREQUENCY:** _____ x/day

SPECIAL PROTOCOLS/NOTES: Do not slouch. _____

_____

_____

_____

PATIENT NAME: _____ DATE: _____

THERAPIST NAME: _____

Sitting Shoulder
Internal Rotation

PURPOSE: To strengthen shoulder muscles.

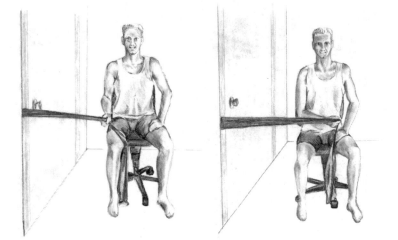

INSTRUCTION: Tie knot in one end of resistive band and shut knot in door. Sit in neutral position with right side of body toward door. Grasp other end of band with right hand. Bend right elbow and bring hand in toward abdomen. Repeat with opposite side.

HOLD: _____ second(s) **REPEAT:** _____ time(s) **FREQUENCY:** _____ x/day

SPECIAL PROTOCOLS/NOTES: Do not slouch. _____

_____

_____

_____

PATIENT NAME: _____ DATE: _____

THERAPIST NAME: _____

Sitting Unilateral Shoulder External Rotation

PURPOSE: To strengthen shoulder muscles.

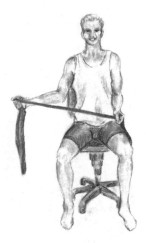

INSTRUCTION: Wrap ends of resistive band around each hand. Sit in neutral position. Bend elbows. Begin with right hand next to abdomen. Move hand away from abdomen holding left hand close to body. Repeat with opposite side.

HOLD: _____ second(s) **REPEAT:** _____ time(s) **FREQUENCY:** _____ x/day

SPECIAL PROTOCOLS/NOTES: Do not slouch. _____
_____
_____
_____

PATIENT NAME: _____   DATE: _____
THERAPIST NAME: _____

Sitting Bilateral Shoulder External Rotation

PURPOSE: To strengthen shoulder muscles.

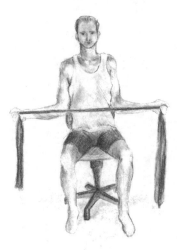

INSTRUCTION: Wrap ends of resistive band around each hand. Sit in neutral position. Bend both elbows placing hands next to abdomen. Move hands away from abdomen keeping elbows next to body. Return to starting position.

HOLD: _____ second(s) **REPEAT:** _____ time(s) **FREQUENCY:** _____ x/day

SPECIAL PROTOCOLS/NOTES: <u>Do not slouch.</u>
_____
_____
_____

PATIENT NAME: _____ DATE: _____

THERAPIST NAME: _____

Sitting Unilateral Protraction

PURPOSE: To strengthen chest and shoulder muscles.

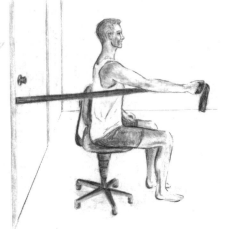

INSTRUCTION: Tie knot in one end of resistive band and shut knot in door at elbow height. Sit in neutral position with back to door. Wrap other end of band around right hand. Bend right elbow and place next to side of body. Push hand forward. Return to starting position. Repeat with opposite side.

HOLD: _____ second(s) **REPEAT:** _____ time(s) **FREQUENCY:** _____ x/day

SPECIAL PROTOCOLS/NOTES: Do not round shoulders. _____

_____

_____

_____

VARIATION: Tie knot in middle of resistive band and shut knot in door at elbow height. Wrap ends of resistive band around each hand. Bend elbows and push both hands forward together.

PATIENT NAME: _____ DATE: _____

THERAPIST NAME: _____

Sitting Bilateral Shoulder Protraction

PURPOSE: To strengthen shoulder muscles.

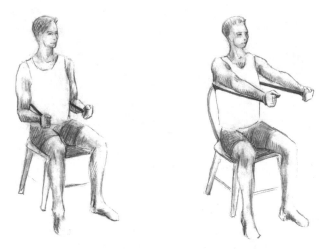

INSTRUCTION: Sit in neutral position. Wrap ends of resistive band around each hand. Loop band behind back. Bend both elbows and push hands forward.

HOLD: _____ second(s) **REPEAT:** _____ time(s) **FREQUENCY:** _____ x/day

SPECIAL PROTOCOLS/NOTES: Do not round shoulders.

_____

_____

_____

VARIATION: Follow instructions as above, however, push only one hand forward at a time.

PATIENT NAME: _____   DATE: _____

THERAPIST NAME: _____

Sitting Unilateral Shoulder Rowing

PURPOSE: To strengthen arm, shoulder, and mid-back muscles.

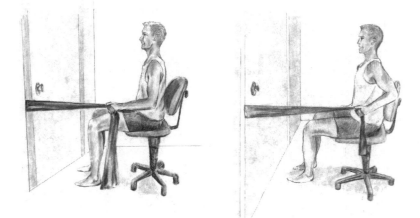

INSTRUCTION: Tie knot in one end of resistive band and shut knot in door. Sit in neutral position, facing door. Wrap other end of band around left hand. Bend left elbow. Pull elbow back. Repeat with opposite side.

HOLD: _____ second(s) **REPEAT:** _____ time(s) **FREQUENCY:** _____ x/day

SPECIAL PROTOCOLS/NOTES: Do not slouch. _____
_____
_____
_____

PATIENT NAME: _____ DATE: _____

THERAPIST NAME: _____

Sitting Bilateral Shoulder Rowing

PURPOSE: To strengthen arm, shoulder, and mid-back muscles.

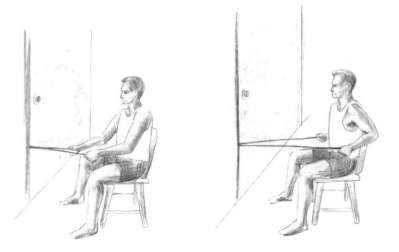

INSTRUCTION: Tie knot in middle of resistive band and shut knot in door. Sit in neutral position, facing door. Grasp ends of resistive band with both hands. Bend elbows. Pull both elbows back.

HOLD: _____ second(s) **REPEAT:** _____ time(s) **FREQUENCY:** _____ x/day

SPECIAL PROTOCOLS/NOTES: <u>Do not slouch.</u>

_____

_____

_____

PATIENT NAME: _____ DATE: _____

THERAPIST NAME: _____

Sitting Upright Row

PURPOSE: To strengthen shoulder and mid-back muscles.

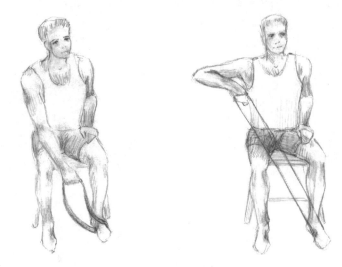

INSTRUCTION: Loop resistive band under left foot and grasp both ends of band with right hand. Sit in neutral position. Reach right hand toward opposite foot. Bend elbow and raise to shoulder height. Repeat with opposite side.

HOLD: _____ second(s) **REPEAT:** _____ time(s) **FREQUENCY:** _____ x/day

SPECIAL PROTOCOLS/NOTES: Do not arch or round back. _____

_____

_____

_____

PATIENT NAME: _____	DATE: _____
THERAPIST NAME: _____	

Sitting Bilateral Shoulder Rowing in Trunk Flexion

PURPOSE: To strengthen arm, shoulder, and mid-back muscles.

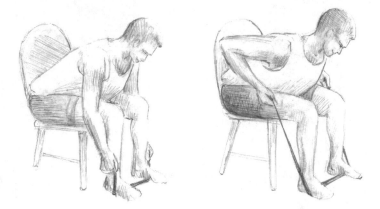

INSTRUCTION: Loop resistive band under both feet. Grasp ends of band with both hands. Sit in neutral position. Lean forward at waist. Bend both elbows. Pull elbows back.

HOLD: _____ second(s) **REPEAT:** _____ time(s) **FREQUENCY:** _____ x/day

SPECIAL PROTOCOLS/NOTES: Do not arch or round back.

_____

_____

_____

VARIATION: Follow directions as above, however, pull only one elbow back at a time.

PATIENT NAME: _____ DATE: _____

THERAPIST NAME: _____

Sitting Bow Exercise

PURPOSE: To strengthen arm and shoulder muscles.

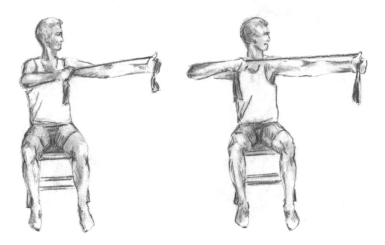

INSTRUCTION: Sit in neutral position with head turned to the left. Wrap ends of resistive band around each hand. Raise left arm out away from body to shoulder height. Rotate left thumb toward ceiling. Bend right elbow and raise to shoulder height. Move right elbow back, keeping elbow at shoulder height. Repeat with opposite side.

HOLD: _____ second(s) **REPEAT:** _____ time(s) **FREQUENCY:** _____ x/day

SPECIAL PROTOCOLS/NOTES: _____
_____
_____
_____

PATIENT NAME: _____ DATE: _____

THERAPIST NAME: _____

Sitting Shoulder PNF Diagonal One — Flexion on Ball

PURPOSE: To strengthen shoulder muscles.

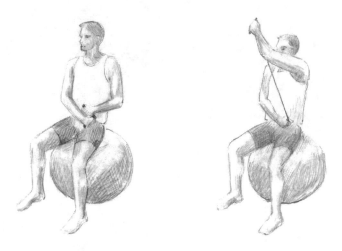

INSTRUCTION: Sit on ball in neutral position. Wrap ends of resistive band around each hand. Place right hand on left hip. Raise left hand up and over right shoulder. Repeat with opposite side.

HOLD: _____ second(s)   **REPEAT:** _____ time(s)   **FREQUENCY:** _____ x/day

SPECIAL PROTOCOLS/NOTES: Do not round shoulders. _____
_____
_____
_____

PATIENT NAME: _____   DATE: _____

THERAPIST NAME: _____

Sitting Shoulder PNF Diagonal Two — Flexion on Ball

PURPOSE: To strengthen shoulder muscles.

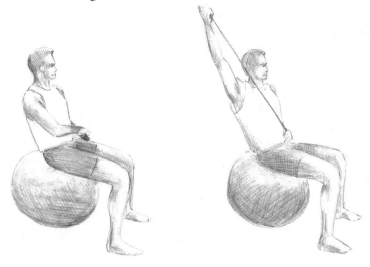

INSTRUCTION: Sit in neutral position. Wrap ends of resistive band around each hand. Place right hand on left hip. Raise right arm up and overhead. Repeat with opposite side.

HOLD: _____ second(s) **REPEAT:** _____ time(s) **FREQUENCY:** _____ x/day

SPECIAL PROTOCOLS/NOTES: Do not round shoulders. _____
_____
_____
_____

PATIENT NAME: _____ DATE: _____

THERAPIST NAME: _____

Sitting Shoulder PNF Diagonal One — Extension on Ball

PURPOSE: To strengthen arm, shoulder, and trunk muscles and improve balance reactions.

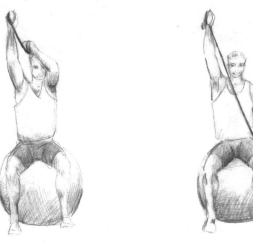

INSTRUCTION: Sit on ball in neutral position. Grasp ends of resistive band with both hands. Raise both arms overhead. Place left hand next to right elbow. Pull left hand down to left side of hip. Repeat with opposite side.

HOLD: _____ second(s) **REPEAT:** _____ time(s) **FREQUENCY:** _____ x/day

SPECIAL PROTOCOLS/NOTES: Do not round shoulders. _____

_____

_____

_____

PATIENT NAME: _____ DATE: _____

THERAPIST NAME: _____

Sitting Shoulder PNF Diagonal Two — Extension on Ball

PURPOSE: To strengthen arm, shoulder, and trunk muscles and improve balance reactions.

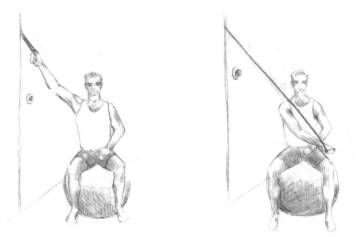

INSTRUCTION: Tie knot in one end of resistive band and shut knot in door. Sit in neutral position on ball with right side of body toward door. Grasp other end of band with right hand. Raise right arm overhead. Pull right hand down to left side of hip. Repeat with opposite side.

HOLD: _____ second(s) **REPEAT:** _____ time(s) **FREQUENCY:** _____ x/day

SPECIAL PROTOCOLS/NOTES: Do not round shoulders. _____
_____
_____
_____

PATIENT NAME: _____ DATE: _____

THERAPIST NAME: _____

Sitting Abdominal Oblique
Sit Back on Ball

PURPOSE: To strengthen oblique abdominal, arm, and shoulder muscles.

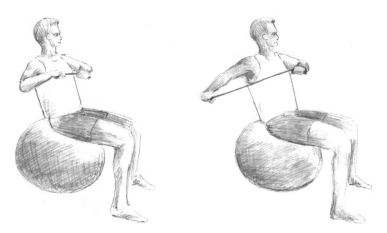

INSTRUCTION: Sit on ball in neutral position. Wrap ends of resistive band around each hand. Lean back on ball. Bend elbows and raise to shoulder height. Extend right arm out to side of body. Return to starting position. Repeat with opposite side.

HOLD: _____ second(s) **REPEAT:** _____ time(s) **FREQUENCY:** _____ x/day

SPECIAL PROTOCOLS/NOTES: Do not bend at waist. Do not arch back.

_____

_____

_____

PATIENT NAME: _____ DATE: _____

THERAPIST NAME: _____

Sitting Trunk Flexion

PURPOSE: To strengthen abdominal and neck muscles.

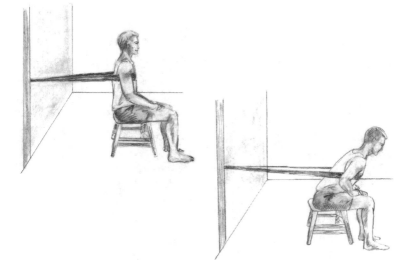

INSTRUCTION: Tie ends of resistive band together and shut knot in door. Sit in chair in neutral position, facing away from door. Loop band around chest. Lean forward at the waist. Keep back straight. Return to starting position.

HOLD: _____ second(s) **REPEAT:** _____ time(s) **FREQUENCY:** _____ x/day

SPECIAL PROTOCOLS/NOTES: Do not slouch.
_____
_____
_____

PATIENT NAME: _____   DATE: _____
THERAPIST NAME: _____

Sitting Trunk Extension

PURPOSE: To strengthen back and neck muscles.

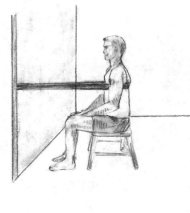
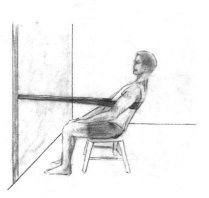

INSTRUCTION: Tie ends of resistive band together and shut knot in door. Sit in chair in neutral position, facing door. Loop band around back. Lean backward keeping back straight. Return to starting position.

HOLD: _____ second(s) **REPEAT:** _____ time(s) **FREQUENCY:** _____ x/day

SPECIAL PROTOCOLS/NOTES: Do not slouch. _____
_____
_____
_____

PATIENT NAME: _____ DATE: _____
THERAPIST NAME: _____

Sitting Trunk Side Bend

PURPOSE: To strengthen side trunk muscles.

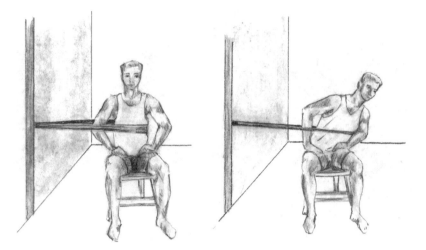

INSTRUCTION: Tie ends of resistive band together and shut knot in door. Sit in chair in neutral position with right side facing door. Loop band around chest. Lean to the left bending at the waist. Return to starting position. Repeat with opposite side.

HOLD: _____ second(s) **REPEAT:** _____ time(s) **FREQUENCY:** _____ x/day

SPECIAL PROTOCOLS/NOTES: Do not slouch. _____
_____
_____
_____

PATIENT NAME: _____ DATE: _____

THERAPIST NAME: _____

Sitting Trunk Rotation

PURPOSE: To strengthen abdominal and trunk muscles.

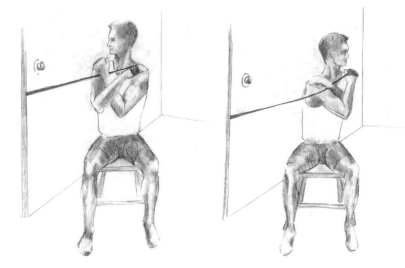

INSTRUCTION: Tie knot in one end of resistive band and shut knot in door. Wrap other end of band around left hand. Sit in chair in neutral position with right side facing door. Rotate trunk and head toward door. Rotate trunk and head away from door. Repeat with opposite side.

HOLD: _____ second(s) **REPEAT:** _____ time(s) **FREQUENCY:** _____ x/day

SPECIAL PROTOCOLS/NOTES: Do not rotate hips with upper body. Keep hips facing forward and arms close to body. _____

PATIENT NAME: _____ DATE: _____

THERAPIST NAME: _____

Sitting Hip Flexion

PURPOSE: To strengthen hip muscles.

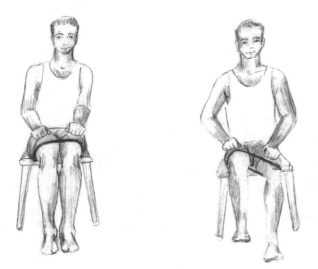

INSTRUCTION: Sit in chair in neutral position. Tie ends of resistive band together. Loop band around both knees. Raise right knee toward ceiling. Repeat with opposite side.

HOLD: _____ second(s) **REPEAT:** _____ time(s) **FREQUENCY:** _____ x/day

SPECIAL PROTOCOLS/NOTES: _____

_____

_____

_____

PATIENT NAME: _____ DATE: _____

THERAPIST NAME: _____

Sitting Hip Extension

PURPOSE: To strengthen hip muscles.

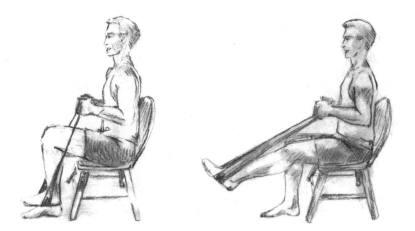

INSTRUCTION: Sit in chair in neutral position. Grasp ends of resistive band with both hands. Loop band around left foot. Raise left knee toward ceiling. Straighten knee and push foot toward floor. Repeat with opposite side.

HOLD: _____ second(s) **REPEAT:** _____ time(s) **FREQUENCY:** _____ x/day

SPECIAL PROTOCOLS/NOTES: _____

_____

_____

_____

PATIENT NAME: _____ DATE: _____

THERAPIST NAME: _____

Sitting Hip Abduction

PURPOSE: To strengthen outer thigh muscles.

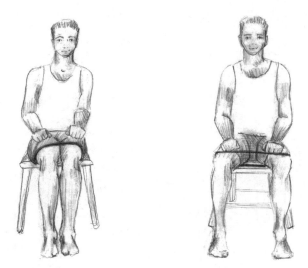

INSTRUCTION: Sit in chair in neutral position. Loop resistive band around both thighs. Move right knee away from body and return to starting position. Repeat with opposite side.

HOLD: _____ second(s) **REPEAT:** _____ time(s) **FREQUENCY:** _____ x/day

SPECIAL PROTOCOLS/NOTES: Do not slouch. _____
_____
_____
_____

PATIENT NAME: _____ DATE: _____

THERAPIST NAME: _____

Sitting Hip Adduction

PURPOSE: To strengthen inner thigh muscles.

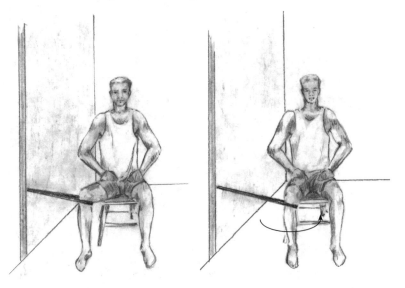

INSTRUCTION: Tie ends of resistive band together and shut knot in door. Sit in chair in neutral position with right side facing door and right knee away from body, close to door. Loop band around right knee. Move knee in and touch left knee. Return to starting position. Repeat with opposite side.

HOLD: _____ second(s) **REPEAT:** _____ time(s) **FREQUENCY:** _____ x/day

SPECIAL PROTOCOLS/NOTES: Do not slouch. _____
_____
_____
_____

PATIENT NAME: _____ DATE: _____
THERAPIST NAME: _____

Sitting Hip Adduction/Abduction with Small Ball

PURPOSE: To strengthen inner and outer thigh muscles.

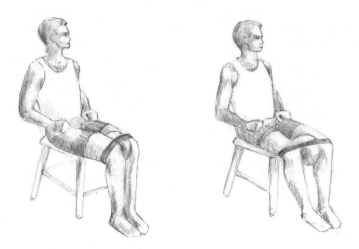

INSTRUCTION: Tie ends of resistive band together. Loop band around both thighs and place small ball between knees. Sit in chair in a reclined position with pillow behind back and heels together. Press knees into ball. Hold _____ second(s). Move knees apart without moving feet.

REPEAT: _____ time(s)   **FREQUENCY:** _____ x/day

SPECIAL PROTOCOLS/NOTES: Maintain neutral position. Do not hold breath. _____

_____

_____

PATIENT NAME: _____ DATE: _____

THERAPIST NAME: _____

Sitting Hip Adduction and Abduction with Small Ball While Doing Kegel Exercise

PURPOSE: To strengthen inner and outer thigh and pelvic floor muscles.

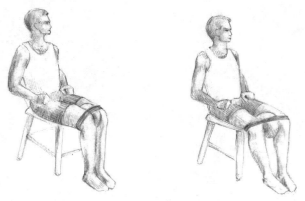

INSTRUCTION: Tie ends of resistive band together. Loop band around both thighs and place small ball between knees. Sit in chair in a reclined position with pillow behind back and heels together. Gently press knees into ball while tightening pelvic floor muscles for _____ second(s). Slowly relax pelvic floor muscles and knees. Move knees apart without moving feet.

REPEAT: _____ time(s)   **FREQUENCY:** _____ x/day

SPECIAL PROTOCOLS/NOTES: Maintain neutral position. Do not hold breath.

_____

_____

PATIENT NAME: _____ DATE: _____

THERAPIST NAME: _____

Sitting Hip Internal Rotation

PURPOSE: To strengthen buttock and hip muscles.

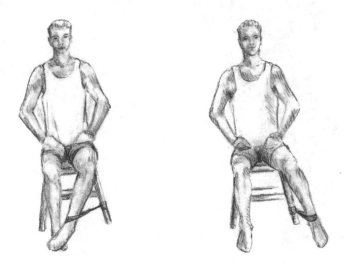

INSTRUCTION: Sit in neutral position. Tie resistive band around left chair leg and loop around left ankle. Begin with left foot touching right foot. Move left foot out away from side of chair, without moving knee. Repeat with opposite side.

HOLD: _____ second(s) **REPEAT:** _____ time(s) **FREQUENCY:** _____ x/day

SPECIAL PROTOCOLS/NOTES: _____
_____
_____
_____

PATIENT NAME: _____ DATE: _____

THERAPIST NAME: _____

Sitting Hip External Rotation

PURPOSE: To strengthen buttock and hip muscles.

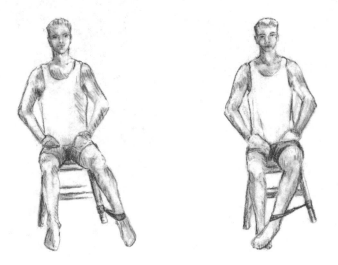

INSTRUCTION: Sit in chair in neutral position. Tie resistive band around left chair leg and loop around ankle. Begin with left foot out away from side of chair. Move left foot in and touch right foot, without moving knee. Repeat with opposite side.

HOLD: _____ second(s) **REPEAT:** _____ time(s) **FREQUENCY:** _____ x/day

SPECIAL PROTOCOLS/NOTES: _____

_____

_____

_____

PATIENT NAME: _____ DATE: _____

THERAPIST NAME: _____

Sitting Knee Flexion

PURPOSE: To strengthen back of thigh muscles.

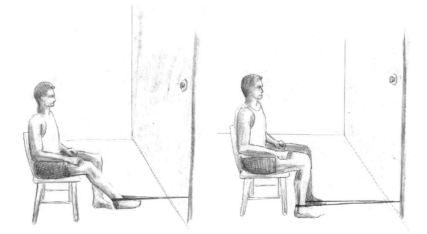

INSTRUCTION: Tie ends of resistive band together and shut knot in door. Loop band around right ankle. Sit in chair in neutral position, facing door with right knee straight. Bend knee back toward chair. Repeat with opposite side.

HOLD: _____ second(s) **REPEAT:** _____ time(s) **FREQUENCY:** _____ x/day

SPECIAL PROTOCOLS/NOTES: _____

_____

_____

_____

PATIENT NAME: _____ DATE: _____

THERAPIST NAME: _____

Sitting Knee Extension

PURPOSE: To strengthen front of thigh muscles.

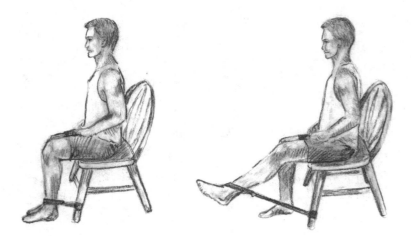

INSTRUCTION: Sit in chair in neutral position. Tie resistive band around right chair leg and loop around right ankle. Straighten knee. Repeat with opposite side.

HOLD: _____ second(s) **REPEAT:** _____ time(s) **FREQUENCY:** _____ x/day

SPECIAL PROTOCOLS/NOTES: _____

_____

_____

_____

PATIENT NAME: _____ DATE: _____

THERAPIST NAME: _____

Sitting Vastus Medialis Obliques Exercise on Ball

PURPOSE: To strengthen knee and thigh muscles.

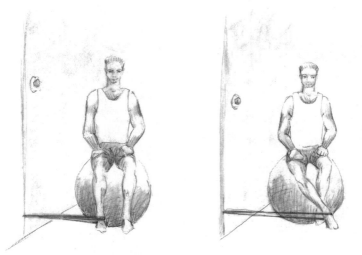

INSTRUCTION: Tie ends of resistive band together and shut knot in door. Sit on ball in neutral position with right side of body facing door. Loop band around right ankle. Cross right foot over left foot. Repeat with opposite side.

HOLD: _____ second(s) **REPEAT:** _____ time(s) **FREQUENCY:** _____ x/day

SPECIAL PROTOCOLS/NOTES: _____
_____
_____
_____

PATIENT NAME: _____ DATE: _____

THERAPIST NAME: _____

Sitting Plantarflexion

PURPOSE: To strengthen calf muscles.

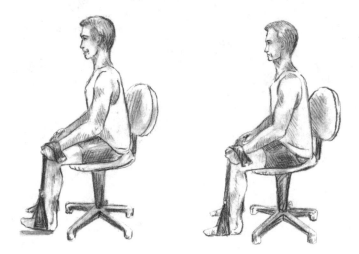

INSTRUCTION: Sit in chair in neutral position. Grasp ends of resistive band in left hand. Loop band around ball of left foot. Pull toes up and push toes down. Repeat with opposite side.

HOLD: _____ second(s) **REPEAT:** _____ time(s) **FREQUENCY:** _____ x/day

SPECIAL PROTOCOLS/NOTES: <u>Keep heel on floor.</u> _____

_____

_____

_____

PATIENT NAME: _____   DATE: _____

THERAPIST NAME: _____

Sitting Plantarflexion with Foot on Book

PURPOSE: To strengthen calf muscles.

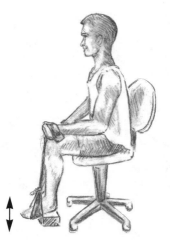

INSTRUCTION: Sit in chair in neutral position with left heel on book. Grasp ends of resistive band in left hand. Loop band around ball of left foot. Pull toes up and push toes down toward floor. Repeat with opposite side.

HOLD: _____ second(s) **REPEAT:** _____ time(s) **FREQUENCY:** _____ x/day

SPECIAL PROTOCOLS/NOTES: Keep heel on book. _____

_____

_____

_____

PATIENT NAME: _____   DATE: _____

THERAPIST NAME: _____

Sitting Dorsiflexion

PURPOSE: To strengthen calf muscles.

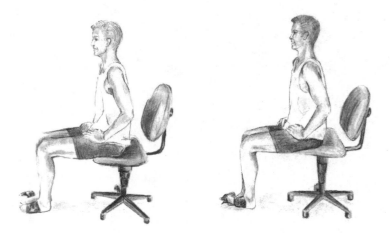

INSTRUCTION: Sit in chair in neutral position. Loop resistive band around left foot. Step on band with right foot. Raise left foot up toward ceiling. Repeat with opposite foot.

HOLD: _____ second(s) **REPEAT:** _____ time(s) **FREQUENCY:** _____ x/day

SPECIAL PROTOCOLS/NOTES: Keep heel on floor. _____

_____

_____

_____

PATIENT NAME: _____ DATE: _____

THERAPIST NAME: _____

Sitting Inversion

PURPOSE: To strengthen inner ankle and leg muscles.

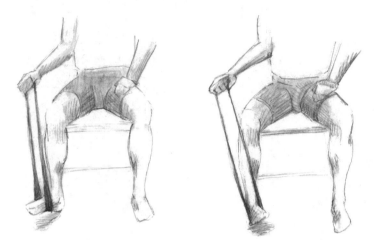

INSTRUCTION: Sit in neutral position. Loop resistive band around right foot. Grasp ends of band in right hand. Raise right toes up and out. Move right toes up and in. Repeat with opposite side.

HOLD: _____ second(s) **REPEAT:** _____ time(s) **FREQUENCY:** _____ x/day

SPECIAL PROTOCOLS/NOTES: Keep heel on floor. _____

_____

_____

_____

PATIENT NAME: _____ DATE: _____

THERAPIST NAME: _____

Sitting Eversion

PURPOSE: To strengthen outer ankle and leg muscles.

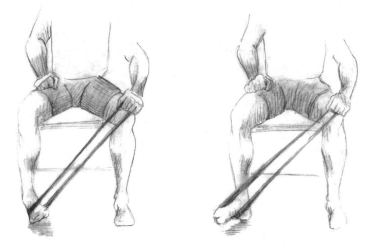

INSTRUCTION: Sit in neutral position. Loop resistive band around right foot. Grasp ends of band in left hand and rest on outside of left knee. Raise right toes up and in. Move toes up and out. Repeat with opposite side.

HOLD: _____ second(s) **REPEAT:** _____ time(s) **FREQUENCY:** _____ x/day

SPECIAL PROTOCOLS/NOTES: Keep heel on floor.
_____
_____
_____
_____

PATIENT NAME: _____ DATE: _____

THERAPIST NAME: _____

Long Sitting Tricep Lift

PURPOSE: To strengthen back of arm and wrist muscles.

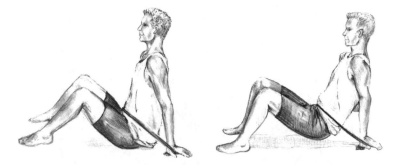

INSTRUCTION: Sit in neutral position with knees bent. Wrap ends of resistive band around each hand. Loop band around waist. Lift buttocks four inches off floor.

HOLD: _____ second(s) **REPEAT:** _____ time(s) **FREQUENCY:** _____ x/day

SPECIAL PROTOCOLS/NOTES: _____

_____

_____

_____

PATIENT NAME: _____ DATE: _____

THERAPIST NAME: _____

Long Sitting Tricep Lift with Leg Lift

PURPOSE: To strengthen back of arm, leg and wrist muscles.

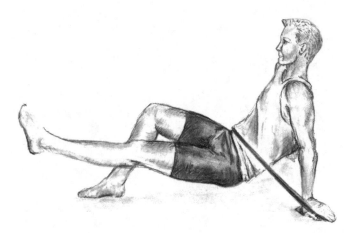

INSTRUCTION: Sit in neutral position with one knee bent and one knee straight. Wrap ends of resistive band around each hand. Loop band around waist. Lift right buttock four inches off floor as straight right leg is raised. Repeat with opposite side.

HOLD: _____ second(s) **REPEAT:** _____ time(s) **FREQUENCY:** _____ x/day

SPECIAL PROTOCOLS/NOTES: _____

_____

_____

_____

PATIENT NAME: _____ DATE: _____

THERAPIST NAME: _____

Long Sitting Unilateral Shoulder Rowing

PURPOSE: To strengthen arm and mid-back muscles.

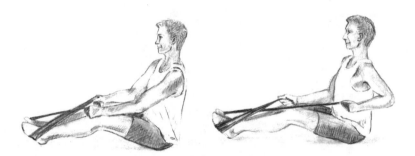

INSTRUCTION: Sit in neutral position with legs straight out in front of body. Grasp ends of resistive band with both hands. Loop band around both forefeet. Pull left elbow back. Repeat with opposite side.

HOLD: _____ second(s) **REPEAT:** _____ time(s) **FREQUENCY:** _____ x/day

SPECIAL PROTOCOLS/NOTES: Do not lift shoulders. _____

_____

_____

_____

PATIENT NAME: _____   DATE: _____

THERAPIST NAME: _____

Long Sitting Bilateral Shoulder Rowing

PURPOSE: To strengthen arm and mid-back muscles.

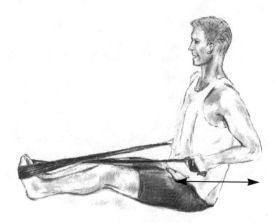

INSTRUCTION: Sit in neutral position with legs straight out in front of body. Grasp ends of band with both hands. Loop band around both forefeet. Pull both elbows back.

HOLD: _____ second(s) **REPEAT:** _____ time(s) **FREQUENCY:** _____ x/day

SPECIAL PROTOCOLS/NOTES: Do not lift shoulders. _____

_____

_____

_____

PATIENT NAME: _____ DATE: _____

THERAPIST NAME: _____

Long Sitting Ankle Plantarflexion

PURPOSE: To strengthen calf muscles.

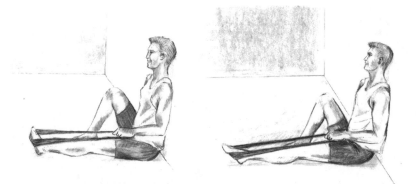

INSTRUCTION: Sit in neutral position with back against wall with right knee bent and left knee straight. Grasp ends of resistive band with left hand. Loop band around left forefoot. Push toes down to floor. Repeat with opposite side.

HOLD: _____ second(s) **REPEAT:** _____ time(s) **FREQUENCY:** _____ x/day

SPECIAL PROTOCOLS/NOTES: Keep heel on floor.
_____
_____
_____

PATIENT NAME: _____ DATE: _____

THERAPIST NAME: _____

Long Sitting Ankle Dorsiflexion

PURPOSE: To strengthen shin muscles.

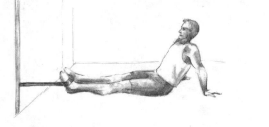

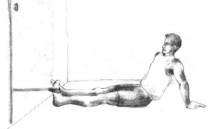

INSTRUCTION: Sit on floor with legs out straight and arms behind back, facing door. Tie ends of resistive band together and shut knot in door. Loop band around right forefoot. Point toes toward door. Pull toes up toward nose. Repeat with opposite side.

HOLD: _____ second(s) **REPEAT:** _____ time(s) **FREQUENCY:** _____ x/day

SPECIAL PROTOCOLS/NOTES: Keep heel on floor. _____

_____

_____

_____

PATIENT NAME: _____ DATE: _____

THERAPIST NAME: _____

Long Sitting Ankle Dorsiflexion with Knee Flexion

PURPOSE: To strengthen shin muscles.

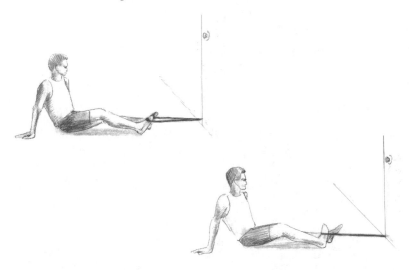

INSTRUCTION: Sit on floor with right knee bent and arms behind back, facing door. Tie ends of resistive band together and shut knot in door. Loop band around right forefoot. Point toes of right foot toward door. Pull toes up toward nose. Repeat with opposite side.

HOLD: _____ second(s) **REPEAT:** _____ time(s) **FREQUENCY:** _____ x/day

SPECIAL PROTOCOLS/NOTES: Keep heel on floor. _____

_____

_____

_____

PATIENT NAME: _____ DATE: _____

THERAPIST NAME: _____

Quadriped and Prone Exercises

CHAPTER FIVE

Quadriped Neutral Position

PURPOSE: To strengthen muscles in an optimal position to avoid injury.

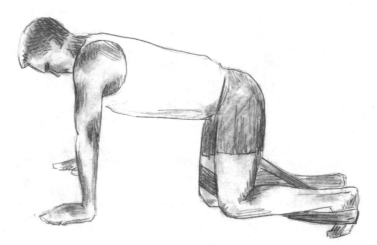

INSTRUCTION: Kneel. Place hands flat on floor. Maintain head alignment with body and natural curve in back.

HOLD: _____ second(s) **REPEAT:** _____ time(s) **FREQUENCY:** _____ x/day

SPECIAL PROTOCOLS/NOTES: Do not round or arch back. _____

_____
_____
_____

PATIENT NAME: _____ DATE: _____

THERAPIST NAME: _____

Quadriped Shoulder Flexion

PURPOSE: To strengthen arm, shoulder, and upper back muscles.

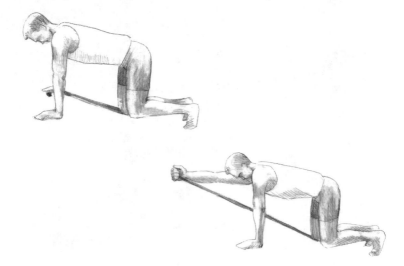

INSTRUCTION: Kneel. Place hands flat on floor. Maintain head alignment with body and natural curve in back. Place resistive band underneath right knee and grasp opposite ends of band with right hand. Raise right arm. Repeat with opposite side.

HOLD: _____ second(s) **REPEAT:** _____ time(s) **FREQUENCY:** _____ x/day

SPECIAL PROTOCOLS/NOTES: Do not round or arch back. _____
_____
_____
_____

PATIENT NAME: _____ DATE: _____
THERAPIST NAME: _____

Quadriped Leg Extension

PURPOSE: To strengthen back, buttock, and leg muscles.

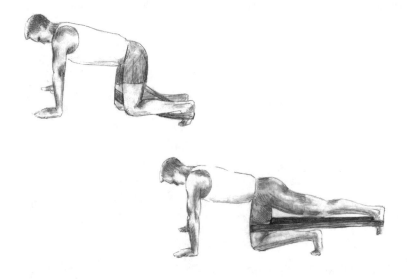

INSTRUCTION: Tie ends of resistive band together. Kneel. Place hands flat on floor. Maintain head alignment with body and natural curve in back. Loop band around right knee and left foot. Extend right leg back. Repeat with opposite side.

HOLD: _____ second(s) **REPEAT:** _____ time(s) **FREQUENCY:** _____ x/day

SPECIAL PROTOCOLS/NOTES: Do not round or arch back. _____

_____

_____

_____

PATIENT NAME: _____ DATE: _____

THERAPIST NAME: _____

Quadriped Shoulder Flexion with Contralateral Leg Extension

PURPOSE: To strengthen arm, back, buttock, leg, and shoulder muscles.

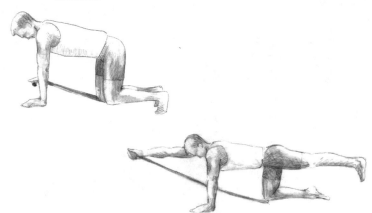

INSTRUCTION: Kneel. Place hands flat on floor. Maintain head alignment with body and natural curve in back. Place one end of resistive band underneath right knee and grasp other end of band with right hand. Raise right arm while extending left leg back. Repeat with opposite side.

HOLD: _____ second(s) **REPEAT:** _____ time(s) **FREQUENCY:** _____ x/day

SPECIAL PROTOCOLS/NOTES: Do not round or arch back.

_____

_____

_____

VARIATION: Follow directions as above, however, loop resistive band around right knee and left foot. Raise right arm while extending right leg back. Repeat with opposite side.

PATIENT NAME: _____ DATE: _____

THERAPIST NAME: _____

Prone Neutral Position

PURPOSE: To strengthen muscles in an optimal position to prevent injury.

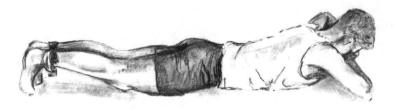

INSTRUCTION: Lie on stomach. Maintain natural curve in back.

HOLD: _____ second(s) **REPEAT:** _____ time(s) **FREQUENCY:** _____ x/day

SPECIAL PROTOCOLS/NOTES: Do not arch back.

_____
_____
_____

PATIENT NAME: _____ DATE: _____
THERAPIST NAME: _____

Prone Mid-Scapular Exercise

PURPOSE: To strengthen mid-back muscles.

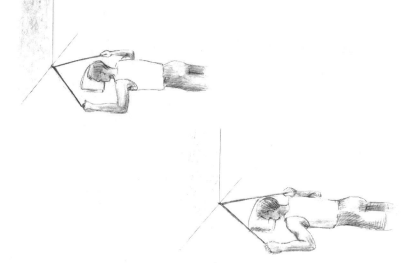

INSTRUCTION: Tie knot in middle of resistive band and shut knot in door. Lie on stomach facing door and place forehead on pillow. Maintain natural curve in back. Raise arms up and grasp ends of band with both hands. Pull shoulder blades down and in toward spine using mid-back muscles. Return to starting position.

HOLD: _____ second(s)   **REPEAT:** _____ time(s) **FREQUENCY:** _____ x/day

SPECIAL PROTOCOLS/NOTES: Do not tighten neck muscles or elevate shoulders when doing exercise.

PATIENT NAME: _____   DATE: _____

THERAPIST NAME: _____

Prone Modified Push-Up

PURPOSE: To strengthen arm, forearm, and shoulder muscles.

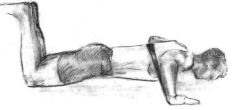

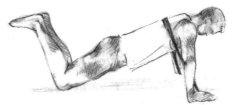

INSTRUCTION: Wrap ends of resistive band around each hand. Loop band behind back. Kneel. Lean forward and place hands on floor. Do a push-up.

HOLD: _____ second(s) **REPEAT:** _____ time(s) **FREQUENCY:** _____ x/day

SPECIAL PROTOCOLS/NOTES: Do not let abdomen sag.

_____

_____

_____

PATIENT NAME: _____ DATE: _____

THERAPIST NAME: _____

Prone Push-Up

PURPOSE: To strengthen arm, forearm, and shoulder muscles.

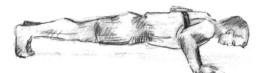

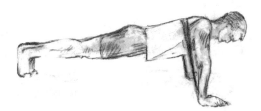

INSTRUCTION: Wrap ends of resistive band around each hand. Loop band behind back. Kneel. Lean forward placing hands on floor and extending legs. Do a push-up.

HOLD: _____ second(s) **REPEAT:** _____ time(s) **FREQUENCY:** _____ x/day

SPECIAL PROTOCOLS/NOTES: Do not let abdomen sag.

_____

_____

_____

PATIENT NAME: _____   DATE: _____

THERAPIST NAME: _____

Prone Shoulder Rowing on Ball

PURPOSE: To strengthen mid-back and shoulder muscles.

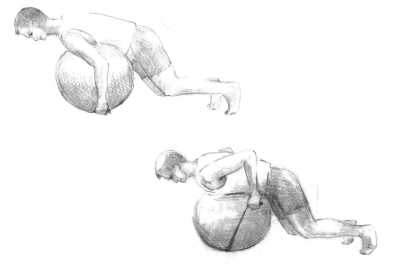

INSTRUCTION: Kneel. Lean forward over ball. Grasp ends of resistive band with both hands. Loop band under ball. Place hands flat on floor next to sides of ball. Bend elbows. Pull elbows up toward ceiling.

HOLD: _____ second(s) **REPEAT:** _____ time(s) **FREQUENCY:** _____ x/day

SPECIAL PROTOCOLS/NOTES: Do not raise shoulders toward ears. Keep back straight throughout exercise. _____

_____

_____

VARIATION: Follow directions as above, however, pull only one elbow up toward ceiling at a time.

PATIENT NAME: _____ DATE: _____

THERAPIST NAME: _____

Prone Trunk Rotation on Ball

PURPOSE: To strengthen arm, mid-back, and shoulder muscles. To improve trunk flexibility.

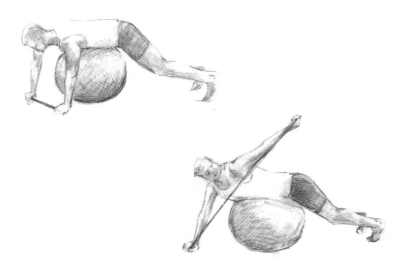

INSTRUCTION: Kneel. Lie with abdomen on ball. Grasp ends of resistive band with both hands. Lift right arm out to side of body. Rotate torso as arm is raised to ceiling. Follow hand motion with eyes, keeping head aligned with body. Repeat with opposite side.

HOLD: _____ second(s) **REPEAT:** _____ time(s) **FREQUENCY:** _____ x/day

SPECIAL PROTOCOLS/NOTES: _____

_____

_____

_____

PATIENT NAME: _____ DATE: _____

THERAPIST NAME: _____

Prone Hip Extension

PURPOSE: To strengthen buttock and thigh muscles.

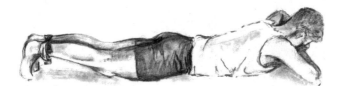

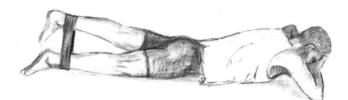

INSTRUCTION: Tie ends of resistive band together. Loop band around both ankles. Lie on stomach in neutral position. Raise left leg up toward ceiling. Repeat with opposite side.

HOLD: _____ second(s) **REPEAT:** _____ time(s) **FREQUENCY:** _____ x/day

SPECIAL PROTOCOLS/NOTES: Do not raise leg so high as to arch back. _____
_____
_____
_____

PATIENT NAME: _____ DATE: _____
THERAPIST NAME: _____

Prone Hip Internal Rotation

PURPOSE: To strengthen inner hip muscles.

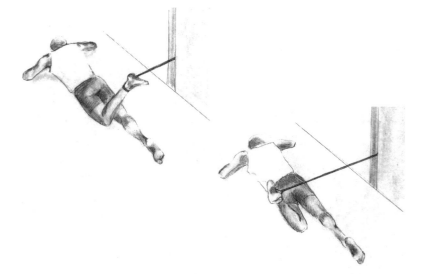

INSTRUCTION: Tie knot in one end of resistive band and shut knot in door at ankle height. Wrap other end of band around left ankle. Lie on stomach. Maintain natural curve in back. Move left ankle out away from door. Repeat with opposite side.

HOLD: _____ second(s) **REPEAT:** _____ time(s) **FREQUENCY:** _____ x/day

SPECIAL PROTOCOLS/NOTES: Do not arch back. _____
_____
_____
_____

PATIENT NAME: _____ DATE: _____

THERAPIST NAME: _____

Prone Hip External Rotation

PURPOSE: To strengthen outer hip muscles.

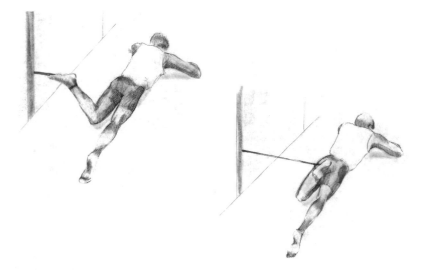

INSTRUCTION: Tie knot in one end of resistive band and shut knot in door at ankle height. Wrap other end of band around left ankle. Lie on stomach. Maintain natural curve in back. Move ankle out away from door. Repeat with opposite side.

HOLD: _____ second(s) **REPEAT:** _____ time(s) **FREQUENCY:** _____ x/day

SPECIAL PROTOCOLS/NOTES: Do not arch back. _____

_____

_____

_____

PATIENT NAME: _____ DATE: _____

THERAPIST NAME: _____

Prone Knee Flexion

PURPOSE: To strengthen back of thigh muscles.

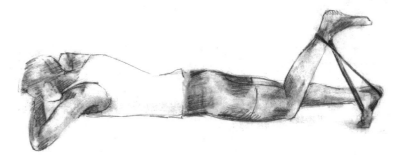

INSTRUCTION: Tie ends of resistive band together. Lie on stomach. Maintain natural curve in back. Loop band around right ankle. Twist band and loop around left ankle. Bend left knee. Repeat with opposite side.

HOLD: _____ second(s) **REPEAT:** _____ time(s) **FREQUENCY:** _____ x/day

SPECIAL PROTOCOLS/NOTES: Do not arch back. _____

_____

_____

_____

PATIENT NAME: _____   DATE: _____

THERAPIST NAME: _____

191

Prone Knee Flexion in Bed

PURPOSE: To strengthen back of thigh muscles.

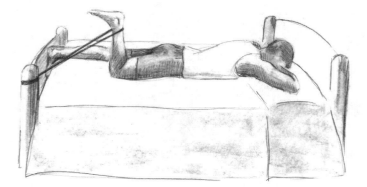

INSTRUCTION: Tie resistive band around bedpost. Lie in bed on stomach. Maintain natural curve in back. Loop band around right ankle. Bend right knee. Repeat with opposite side.

HOLD: _____ second(s) **REPEAT:** _____ time(s) **FREQUENCY:** _____ x/day

SPECIAL PROTOCOLS/NOTES: Do not arch back. _____

_____

_____

_____

PATIENT NAME: _____ DATE: _____

THERAPIST NAME: _____

Prone Knee Extension

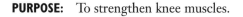

PURPOSE: To strengthen knee muscles.

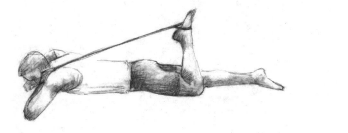

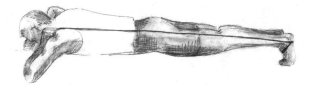

INSTRUCTION: Tie resistive band around left ankle. Lie on stomach in neutral position. Grasp other end of band in left hand. Bend left knee. Straighten knee. Repeat with opposite side.

HOLD: _____ second(s) **REPEAT:** _____ time(s) **FREQUENCY:** _____ x/day

SPECIAL PROTOCOLS/NOTES: Do not bend knee so far as to arch back.

_____

_____

_____

PATIENT NAME: _____ DATE: _____

THERAPIST NAME: _____

CHAPTER SIX

Sidelying Exercises

CHAPTER SIX

Sidelying Neutral Position

PURPOSE: To strengthen muscles in an optimal position to avoid injury.

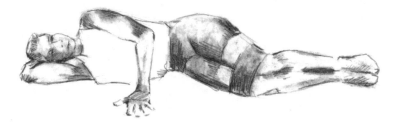

INSTRUCTION: Lie on side with legs slightly bent. Place arm, shoulder, or pillow under head. Maintain natural curve in back.

HOLD: _____ second(s) **REPEAT:** _____ time(s) **FREQUENCY:** _____ x/day

SPECIAL PROTOCOLS/NOTES: _____
_____
_____
_____

PATIENT NAME: _____ DATE: _____

THERAPIST NAME: _____

Sidelying Hip Flexion in Bed

PURPOSE: To strengthen front of thigh muscles.

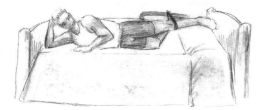

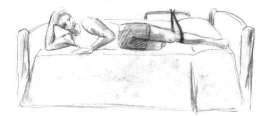

INSTRUCTION: Tie both ends of resistive band to bed rail. Lie on side in bed in neutral position, facing away from bed rail. Loop band below knee. Straighten top leg and place behind bottom leg. Move leg forward. Repeat on opposite side.

HOLD: _____ second(s) **REPEAT:** _____ time(s) **FREQUENCY:** _____ x/day

SPECIAL PROTOCOLS/NOTES: Keep shoulders and hips aligned throughout exercise. Do not allow hips to roll forward or backward. _____
_____
_____

PATIENT NAME: _____ DATE: _____

THERAPIST NAME: _____

Sidelying Hip Extension in Bed

PURPOSE: To strengthen back of thigh muscles.

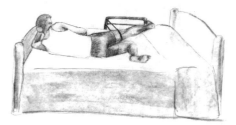

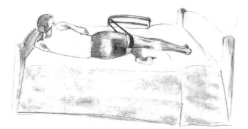

INSTRUCTION: Tie both ends of resistive band to bed rail. Lie on side in bed in neutral position facing bed rail. Loop band around top knee. Straighten top leg and place in front of bottom leg. Move leg backward. Repeat on opposite side.

HOLD: _____ second(s) **REPEAT:** _____ time(s) **FREQUENCY:** _____ x/day

SPECIAL PROTOCOLS/NOTES: Keep shoulders and hips aligned throughout exercise. Do not allow hips to roll forward or backward.

_____

_____

PATIENT NAME: _____ DATE: _____

THERAPIST NAME: _____

Sidelying Hip Abduction

PURPOSE: To strengthen hip and outer thigh muscles.

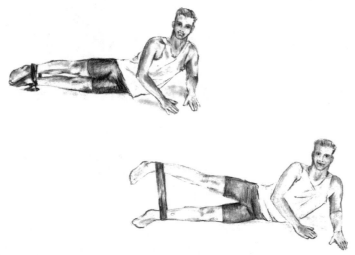

INSTRUCTION: Tie both ends of resistive band together. Loop band around both ankles. Lie on side with both legs straight. Move top foot slightly behind bottom foot. Lift one leg up toward ceiling. Repeat on opposite side.

HOLD: _____ second(s) **REPEAT:** _____ time(s) **FREQUENCY:** _____ x/day

SPECIAL PROTOCOLS/NOTES: _Keep top foot behind bottom leg through-_
out exercise. _____
_____
_____

VARIATIONS: Follow directions as above, however, loop band around legs above knees.

PATIENT NAME: _____ DATE: _____
THERAPIST NAME: _____

Sidelying Hip Abduction with Hip Flexion

PURPOSE: To strengthen buttock and outer thigh muscles.

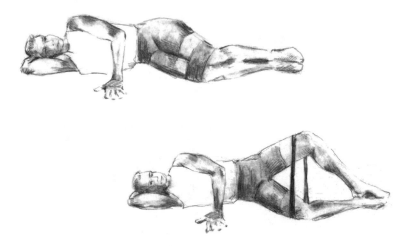

INSTRUCTION: Tie ends of resistive band together. Loop band around thighs. Lie on side in neutral position with both knees bent. Raise both knees up toward ceiling while keeping heels together. Repeat on opposite side.

HOLD: _____ second(s) **REPEAT:** _____ time(s) **FREQUENCY:** _____ x/day

SPECIAL PROTOCOLS/NOTES: Keep shoulders and hips aligned throughout exercise. Do not allow hips to roll backward. _____

_____

_____

PATIENT NAME: _____   DATE: _____

THERAPIST NAME: _____

Sidelying Hip Adduction

PURPOSE: To strengthen inner thigh muscles.

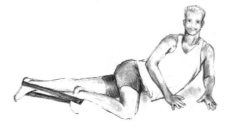

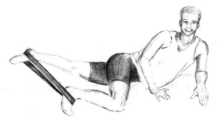

INSTRUCTION: Tie ends of resistive band together. Loop band around both ankles. Lie on side with both legs straight. Bend top knee toward chest. Lift bottom foot up toward ceiling. Repeat on opposite side.

HOLD: _____ second(s) **REPEAT:** _____ time(s) **FREQUENCY:** _____ x/day

SPECIAL PROTOCOLS/NOTES: _____

_____

_____

_____

PATIENT NAME: _____ DATE: _____

THERAPIST NAME: _____

Sidelying Hip Adduction/ Abduction with Small Ball

PURPOSE: To strengthen inner and outer thigh muscles.

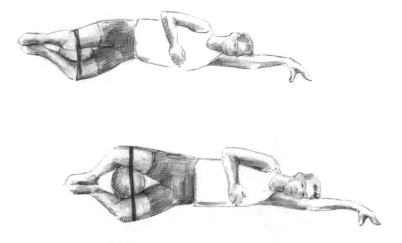

INSTRUCTION: Tie ends of resistive band together. Loop band around both thighs and place small ball between knees. Lie on side in neutral position with both knees bent. Press top knee into ball. Raise top knee up toward ceiling while keeping heels together. Repeat on opposite side.

HOLD: _____ second(s) **REPEAT:** _____ time(s) **FREQUENCY:** _____ x/day

SPECIAL PROTOCOLS/NOTES: Keep shoulders and hips aligned throughout exercise. Do not allow hips to roll backward. _____

_____

_____

PATIENT NAME: _____ DATE: _____

THERAPIST NAME: _____

Sidelying Hip Adduction/ Abduction with Small Ball While Doing Kegel Exercise

PURPOSE: To strengthen inner and outer thigh and pelvic floor muscles.

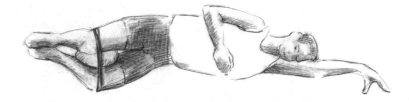

INSTRUCTION: Tie ends of resistive band together. Loop band around both thighs and place small ball between knees. Lie on side in neutral position with both knees bent. Gently press knees into ball while tightening pelvic floor muscles. Hold _____ seconds. Slowly relax pelvic floor muscles and knees. Raise top knee up toward ceiling while keeping heels together. Repeat on opposite side.

HOLD: _____ second(s) **REPEAT:** _____ time(s) **FREQUENCY:** _____ x/day

SPECIAL PROTOCOLS/NOTES: Keep shoulders and hips aligned throughout exercise. Do not allow hips to roll backward. _____

_____

_____

PATIENT NAME: _____ DATE: _____

THERAPIST NAME: _____

CHAPTER SEVEN

Supine
Exercises

CHAPTER SEVEN

Supine Neutral Position

PURPOSE: To strengthen muscles in an optimal position to avoid injury.

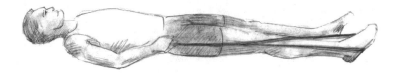

INSTRUCTION: Lie on back. Maintain natural curve in back.

HOLD: _____ second(s) **REPEAT:** _____ time(s) **FREQUENCY:** _____ x/day

SPECIAL PROTOCOLS/NOTES: Do not arch back or flatten back.
_____
_____
_____

PATIENT NAME: _____   DATE: _____

THERAPIST NAME: _____

Supine Shoulder Shrugs in Bed

PURPOSE: To strengthen neck and shoulder muscles.

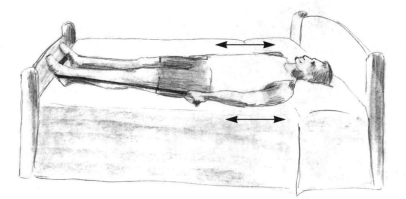

INSTRUCTION: Lie on back in bed in neutral position. Wrap ends of resistive band around each hand. Loop band around both feet. Straighten arms alongside body. Shrug shoulders.

HOLD: _____ second(s) **REPEAT:** _____ time(s) **FREQUENCY:** _____ x/day

SPECIAL PROTOCOLS/NOTES: Do not hold breath.
_____
_____
_____

VARIATION: Follow instructions as above, however, do exercise on floor.

PATIENT NAME: _____ DATE: _____

THERAPIST NAME: _____

Supine Shoulder Flexion

PURPOSE: To strengthen shoulder muscles.

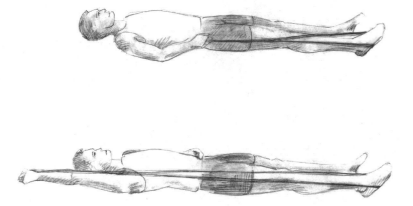

INSTRUCTION: Lie on back in neutral position. Grasp both ends of
resistive band in right hand. Loop band around right
foot. Pull band up overhead. Repeat with opposite side.

HOLD: _____ second(s) **REPEAT:** _____ time(s) **FREQUENCY:** _____ x/day

SPECIAL PROTOCOLS/NOTES: Do not hold breath. _____

_____

_____

_____

PATIENT NAME: _____ DATE: _____

THERAPIST NAME: _____

Supine Shoulder Flexion in Bed

PURPOSE: To strengthen shoulder muscles.

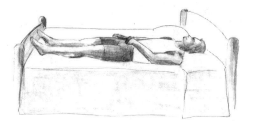

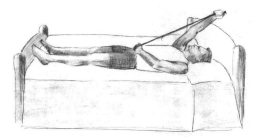

INSTRUCTION: Lie on back in bed in neutral position. Wrap ends of resistive band around each hand. Place both hands on right hip. Raise right arm overhead. Repeat with opposite side.

HOLD: _____ second(s) **REPEAT:** _____ time(s) **FREQUENCY:** _____ x/day

SPECIAL PROTOCOLS/NOTES: Do not hold breath. _____

_____

_____

_____

PATIENT NAME: _____ DATE: _____

THERAPIST NAME: _____

Supine Shoulder Extension

PURPOSE: To strengthen shoulder muscles.

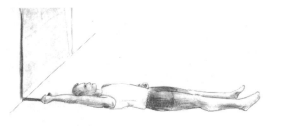

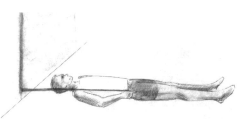

INSTRUCTION: Tie knot in one end of resistive band and shut knot in door. Lie on back, facing away from door in neutral position. Raise right arm overhead and grasp other end of band. Pull band straight down to side of body. Repeat with opposite side.

HOLD: _____ second(s) **REPEAT:** _____ time(s) **FREQUENCY:** _____ x/day

SPECIAL PROTOCOLS/NOTES: Do not hold breath. _____

_____

_____

_____

PATIENT NAME: _____ DATE: _____

THERAPIST NAME: _____

Supine Shoulder Extension in Bed

PURPOSE: To strengthen shoulder muscles.

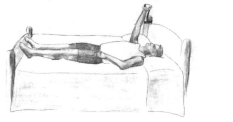

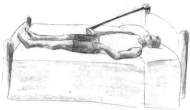

INSTRUCTION: Tie one end of resistive band around bedpost. Lie on back in bed in neutral position. Raise right arm overhead and grasp other end of band. Pull band straight down to side of body. Repeat with opposite side.

HOLD: _____ second(s) **REPEAT:** _____ time(s) **FREQUENCY:** _____ x/day

SPECIAL PROTOCOLS/NOTES: Do not hold breath. _____

_____

_____

_____

PATIENT NAME: _____ DATE: _____

THERAPIST NAME: _____

Supine Shoulder Abduction

PURPOSE: To strengthen shoulder muscles.

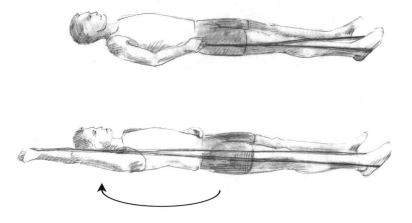

INSTRUCTION: Grasp both ends of resistive band with right hand. Loop band under one foot. Lie on back in bed in neutral position. Slide arm out away from body, and pull band overhead. Repeat with opposite side.

HOLD: _____ second(s) **REPEAT:** _____ time(s) **FREQUENCY:** _____ x/day

SPECIAL PROTOCOLS/NOTES: Do not hold breath. _____

_____

_____

_____

VARIATION: Follow directions as above, however, grasp ends of band with both hands. Loop band under both feet. Slide arms out away from body. Pull band overhead.

PATIENT NAME: _____ DATE: _____

THERAPIST NAME: _____

Supine Shoulder Abduction in Bed

PURPOSE: To strengthen shoulder muscles.

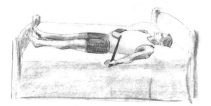

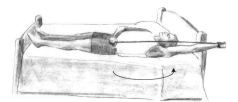

INSTRUCTION: Wrap ends of resistive band around each hand. Lie on back in bed in neutral position. With left hand, pull band overhead from side of body. Return to neutral position. Repeat with opposite side.

HOLD: _____ second(s) **REPEAT:** _____ time(s) **FREQUENCY:** _____ x/day

SPECIAL PROTOCOLS/NOTES: Do not hold breath. _____
_____
_____
_____

PATIENT NAME: _____ DATE: _____
THERAPIST NAME: _____

Supine Shoulder
Horizontal Abduction in Bed

PURPOSE: To strengthen mid-back and shoulder muscles.

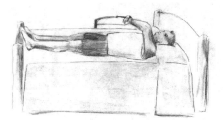

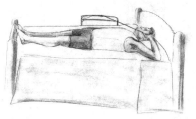

INSTRUCTION: Tie one end of resistive band around bed rail. Wrap other end of band around hand farthest from bed rail. Lie on back in bed in neutral position. Raise arm with band up 90°. Bend elbow and reach hand across chest. Pull elbow back down to side of bed. Repeat with opposite side.

HOLD: _____ second(s) **REPEAT:** _____ time(s) **FREQUENCY:** _____ x/day

SPECIAL PROTOCOLS/NOTES: Do not hold breath.

_____

_____

_____

PATIENT NAME: _____ DATE: _____

THERAPIST NAME: _____

Supine Unilateral Shoulder Adduction

PURPOSE: To strengthen shoulder muscles.

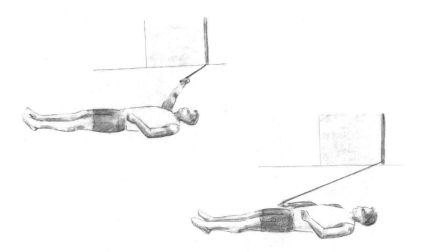

INSTRUCTION: Tie knot in one end of resistive band and shut knot in door. Lie on back in neutral position with right side of body facing door. Raise right arm overhead and grasp other end of band. Pull band down to side of body. Repeat with opposite side.

HOLD: _____ second(s) **REPEAT:** _____ time(s) **FREQUENCY:** _____ x/day

SPECIAL PROTOCOLS/NOTES: Do not hold breath. _____

_____

_____

_____

PATIENT NAME: _____ DATE: _____

THERAPIST NAME: _____

Supine Bilateral Shoulder Adduction

PURPOSE: To strengthen shoulder muscles.

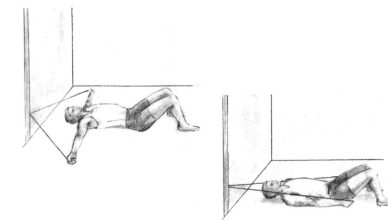

INSTRUCTION: Tie knot in middle of resistive band and shut knot in door. Lie on back in neutral position with knees bent, facing away from door. Raise arms overhead and grasp ends of band with both hands. Pull each end of band down toward sides of body.

HOLD: _____ second(s) **REPEAT:** _____ time(s) **FREQUENCY:** _____ x/day

SPECIAL PROTOCOLS/NOTES: Do not hold breath. _____

_____

_____

_____

PATIENT NAME: _____ DATE: _____

THERAPIST NAME: _____

Supine Horizontal Adduction in Bed

PURPOSE: To strengthen chest and shoulder muscles.

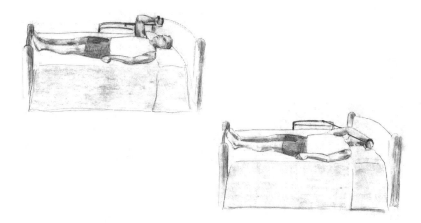

INSTRUCTION: Tie one end of resistive band around bed rail, and wrap other end of band around hand closest to bed rail. Lie on back in bed in neutral position. Raise arm up to 90°. Bend elbow and pull hand across body. Repeat with opposite side.

HOLD: _____ second(s) **REPEAT:** _____ time(s) **FREQUENCY:** _____ x/day

SPECIAL PROTOCOLS/NOTES: Do not hold breath. _____
_____
_____
_____

PATIENT NAME: _____ DATE: _____

THERAPIST NAME: _____

Supine Internal Rotation
in Bed

PURPOSE: To strengthen chest and shoulder muscles.

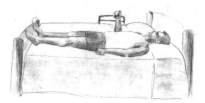

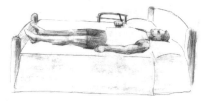

INSTRUCTION: Tie one end of resistive band to bed rail or bedpost. Lie on back in bed in neutral position. Wrap other end of band around hand closest to bed rail. Bend elbow and place against side of body. Pull band toward abdomen. Repeat with opposite side.

HOLD: _____ second(s) **REPEAT:** _____ time(s) **FREQUENCY:** _____ x/day

SPECIAL PROTOCOLS/NOTES: Do not raise elbow off bed.

_____

_____

_____

VARIATION: Follow instructions as above, however, do exercise on floor shutting one end of resistive band in door.

PATIENT NAME: _____ DATE: _____

THERAPIST NAME: _____

Supine Shoulder External Rotation in Bed

PURPOSE: To strengthen mid-back and shoulder muscles.

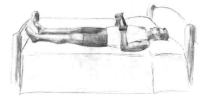

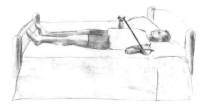

INSTRUCTION: Lie on back in bed in neutral position. Wrap ends of resistive band around each hand. Bend elbows and place against sides of body. Pull hands apart while squeezing shoulder blades together.

HOLD: _____ second(s) **REPEAT:** _____ time(s) **FREQUENCY:** _____ x/day

SPECIAL PROTOCOLS/NOTES: Do not round shoulders. _____

_____

_____

_____

VARIATION: Follow instructions as above, however, do exercise on floor.

PATIENT NAME: _____   DATE: _____

THERAPIST NAME: _____

Supine Shoulder Protraction

PURPOSE: To strengthen shoulder muscles.

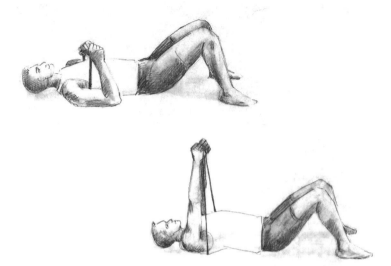

INSTRUCTION: Wrap ends of resistive band around each hand. Loop band behind back. Lie on back in neutral position with knees bent. Bend elbows and push hands toward ceiling.

HOLD: _____ second(s) **REPEAT:** _____ time(s) **FREQUENCY:** _____ x/day

SPECIAL PROTOCOLS/NOTES: Do not round shoulders. _____

_____

_____

_____

VARIATION: Follow instructions as above, however, push only one hand toward ceiling at a time.

PATIENT NAME: _____ DATE: _____

THERAPIST NAME: _____

Supine Shoulder Protraction into Internal Rotation

PURPOSE: To strengthen shoulder muscles.

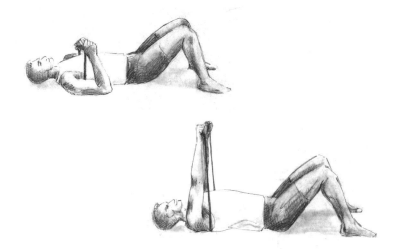

INSTRUCTION: Wrap ends of resistive band around each hand. Loop band behind back. Lie on back in bed in neutral position. Bend elbows and push hands toward ceiling rotating thumbs toward each other.

HOLD: _____ second(s) **REPEAT:** _____ time(s) **FREQUENCY:** _____ x/day

SPECIAL PROTOCOLS/NOTES: Do not round shoulders.

_____

_____

_____

VARIATION: Follow instructions as above, however, push only one hand toward ceiling at a time.

PATIENT NAME: _____ DATE: _____

THERAPIST NAME: _____

Supine Shoulder PNF Diagonal One — Flexion in Bed

PURPOSE: To strengthen shoulder muscles.

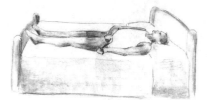

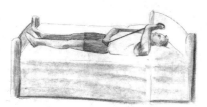

INSTRUCTION: Wrap ends of resistive band around each hand. Lie on back in bed in neutral position. Place right hand on left hip. Raise left hand up and over right shoulder. Repeat with opposite side.

HOLD: _____ second(s) **REPEAT:** _____ time(s) **FREQUENCY:** _____ x/day

SPECIAL PROTOCOLS/NOTES: Do not round shoulders.
_____
_____
_____
_____

PATIENT NAME: _____   DATE: _____

THERAPIST NAME: _____

Supine Shoulder PNF Diagonal Two — Flexion in Bed

PURPOSE: To strengthen shoulder muscles.

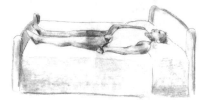

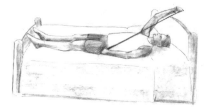

INSTRUCTION: Wrap ends of resistive band around each hand. Lie on back in bed in neutral position. Place right hand on left hip. Raise right hand up and over right shoulder. Repeat with opposite side.

HOLD: _____ second(s) **REPEAT:** _____ time(s) **FREQUENCY:** _____ x/day

SPECIAL PROTOCOLS/NOTES: Do not round shoulders.

_____
_____
_____

PATIENT NAME: _____   DATE: _____

THERAPIST NAME: _____

Supine Shoulder PNF Diagonal One — Extension in Bed

PURPOSE: To strengthen shoulder muscles.

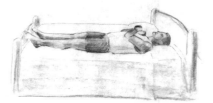

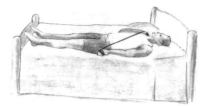

INSTRUCTION: Wrap ends of resistive band around each hand. Lie on back in bed in neutral position. Place both hands on right shoulder. Pull left hand down to left side of hip. Repeat with opposite side.

HOLD: _____ second(s) **REPEAT:** _____ time(s) **FREQUENCY:** _____ x/day

SPECIAL PROTOCOLS/NOTES: Do not round shoulders. _____
_____
_____
_____

PATIENT NAME: _____   DATE: _____

THERAPIST NAME: _____

Supine Shoulder PNF Diagonal Two — Extension in Bed

PURPOSE: To strengthen shoulder muscles.

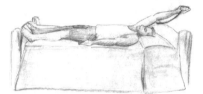

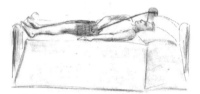

INSTRUCTION: Tie one end of resistive band to bedpost. Grasp other end of band with hand closest to bedpost. Raise right arm overhead. Pull right hand down to left side of hip. Repeat with opposite side.

HOLD: _____ second(s) **REPEAT:** _____ time(s) **FREQUENCY:** _____ x/day

SPECIAL PROTOCOLS/NOTES: Do not round shoulders.

_____
_____
_____

PATIENT NAME: _____ DATE: _____

THERAPIST NAME: _____

Supine Trunk Rotation

PURPOSE: To strengthen oblique abdominal and back muscles.

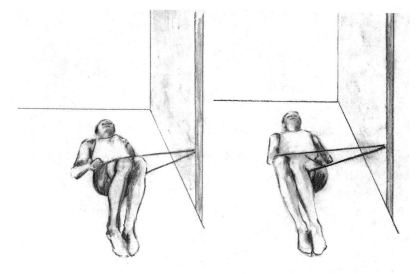

INSTRUCTION: Tie ends of resistive band together and shut knot in door two feet above floor. Loop band around both legs above knees. Lie on back with right side facing door and knees bent. Move knees away from door. Return to starting position. Repeat with opposite side.

HOLD: _____ second(s) **REPEAT:** _____ time(s) **FREQUENCY:** _____ x/day

SPECIAL PROTOCOLS/NOTES: Do not hold breath. _____
_____
_____
_____

PATIENT NAME: _____ DATE: _____

THERAPIST NAME: _____

228

Supine Trunk Counter Rotation

PURPOSE: To strengthen abdominal and trunk muscles.

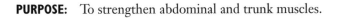

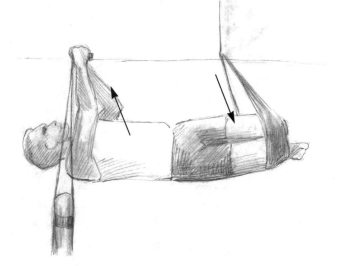

INSTRUCTION: Tie knot in middle of resistive band and shut knot in door two feet above floor. Loop band around legs above knees. Loop second band around bedpost or similar object on opposite side of body; grasp other end of second band with both hands. Lie on back with left side facing door and knees bent. Move knees away from door and hands away from bedpost. Return to starting position. Repeat with bands on opposite side.

HOLD: _____ second(s) **REPEAT:** _____ time(s) **FREQUENCY:** _____ x/day

SPECIAL PROTOCOLS/NOTES: Do not hold breath. _____

_____

_____

_____

PATIENT NAME: _____ DATE: _____

THERAPIST NAME: _____

Supine Abdominal Oblique Curl

PURPOSE: To strengthen oblique muscles in abdomen.

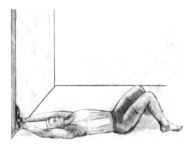

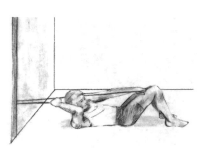

INSTRUCTION: Tie knot in middle of resistive band and shut knot in door two feet above floor. Lie on back with knees bent, facing away from door. Raise arms overhead and grasp ends of resistive band with both hands. Raise head off floor and push left hand toward right knee. Return to starting position. Raise head off floor and push right hand toward left knee.

HOLD: _____ second(s) **REPEAT:** _____ time(s) **FREQUENCY:** _____ x/day

SPECIAL PROTOCOLS/NOTES: Do not hold breath. _____

_____

_____

_____

PATIENT NAME: _____ DATE: _____

THERAPIST NAME: _____

Supine Abdominal Crunch

PURPOSE: To strengthen lower and upper abdominal, arm, and neck muscles.

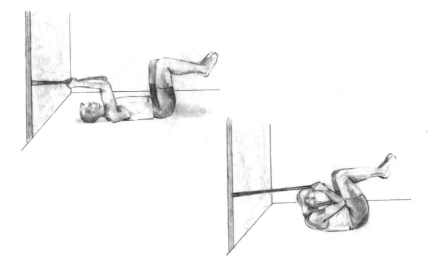

INSTRUCTION: Tie knot in middle of resistive band and shut knot in door two feet above floor. Lie on back with knees bent, facing away from door. Raise arms overhead and grasp ends of band with both hands. Bend knees toward chest, while lifting head, and pulling elbows toward knees. Return to starting position.

HOLD: _____ second(s) **REPEAT:** _____ time(s) **FREQUENCY:** _____ x/day

SPECIAL PROTOCOLS/NOTES: Do not hold breath. _____

_____

_____

_____

PATIENT NAME: _____ DATE: _____

THERAPIST NAME: _____

Supine Lower Abdominal Reverse Curl

PURPOSE: To strengthen lower abdominal muscles.

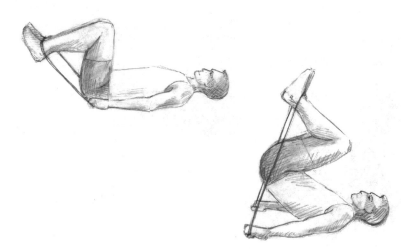

INSTRUCTION: Lie on back with knees bent. Grasp ends of resistive band in both hands. Loop band around both ankles. Place hands at sides of body. Bend knees toward chest, lifting buttocks off floor.

HOLD: _____ second(s) **REPEAT:** _____ time(s) **FREQUENCY:** _____ x/day

SPECIAL PROTOCOLS/NOTES: Do not hold breath. _____

_____

_____

_____

PATIENT NAME: _____ DATE: _____

THERAPIST NAME: _____

Supine Hip Flexion in Bed

PURPOSE: To strengthen abdominal, hip, and thigh muscles.

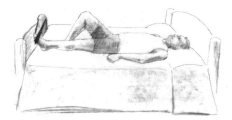

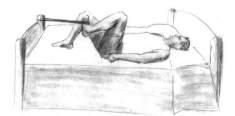

INSTRUCTION: Lie on back in bed in neutral position with right knee bent and left knee straight. Tie ends of resistive band together. Loop band around left foot and bedpost. Bend left knee toward chest. Repeat with opposite side.

HOLD: _____ second(s) **REPEAT:** _____ time(s) **FREQUENCY:** _____ x/day

SPECIAL PROTOCOLS/NOTES: _____

_____

_____

_____

PATIENT NAME: _____ DATE: _____

THERAPIST NAME: _____

Supine Hip Extension in Bed

PURPOSE: To strengthen hip and thigh muscles.

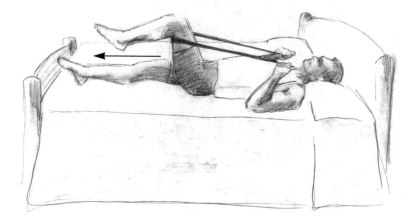

INSTRUCTION: Lie on back in bed in neutral position. Grasp ends of resistive band with both hands. Bend left knee and loop band around left thigh. Straighten hip and knee. Repeat wtih opposite side.

HOLD: _____ second(s) **REPEAT:** _____ time(s) **FREQUENCY:** _____ x/day

SPECIAL PROTOCOLS/NOTES: _____

_____

_____

_____

PATIENT NAME: _____ DATE: _____

THERAPIST NAME: _____

Supine Hip Abduction

PURPOSE: To strengthen hip and outer thigh muscles.

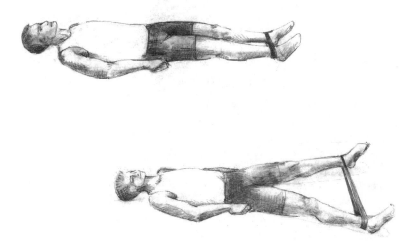

INSTRUCTION: Tie ends of resistive band together. Loop band around both ankles. Lie on back in neutral position. Move legs out away from each other. Return to neutral position.

HOLD: _____ second(s) **REPEAT:** _____ time(s) **FREQUENCY:** _____ x/day

SPECIAL PROTOCOLS/NOTES: _____

_____

_____

_____

VARIATION: Loop band around both ankles. Lie on back in neutral position. Move right leg away from left leg. Repeat with opposite side.

PATIENT NAME: _____ DATE: _____

THERAPIST NAME: _____

Supine Hip Abduction in Bed

PURPOSE: To strengthen hip and outer thigh muscles.

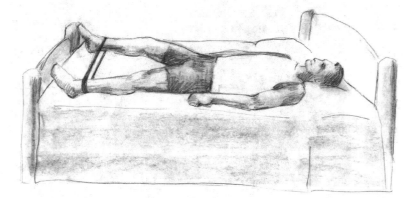

INSTRUCTION: Tie ends of resistive band together. Loop band around both ankles. Lie on back in bed in neutral position. Move legs out away from each other. Return to neutral position.

HOLD: _____ second(s) **REPEAT:** _____ time(s) **FREQUENCY:** _____ x/day

SPECIAL PROTOCOLS/NOTES: _____

_____

_____

_____

VARIATION: Loop band around ankles. Lie on back in neutral position. Move right leg away from left leg. Repeat with left leg moving away from right leg.

PATIENT NAME: _____ DATE: _____

THERAPIST NAME: _____

Supine Hip Abduction in Hooklying Position

PURPOSE: To strengthen hip and outer thigh muscles.

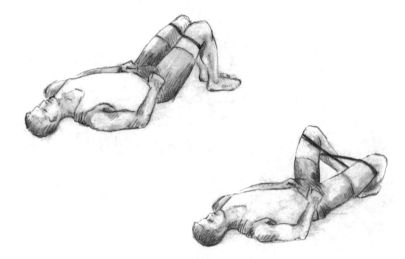

INSTRUCTION: Tie ends of resistive band together. Lie on back in neutral position with knees bent. Slip right leg into loop of resistive band. Twist band and slip left leg into loop of band. Move band up around top of knees. Slowly move knees together and away from each other.

HOLD: _____ second(s) **REPEAT:** _____ time(s) **FREQUENCY:** _____ x/day

SPECIAL PROTOCOLS/NOTES: Do not arch back. Keep abdominal muscles tight throughout exercise.

_____

_____

_____

PATIENT NAME: _____ DATE: _____

THERAPIST NAME: _____

Supine Hip Abduction with Hip and Knee Flexion

PURPOSE: To strengthen abdominal, hip, and inner thigh muscles.

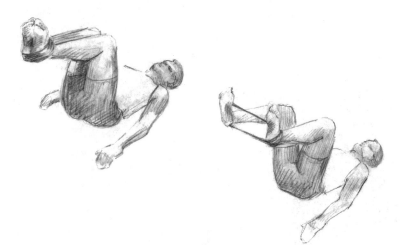

INSTRUCTION: Tie ends of resistive band together. Lie on back in neutral position with knees bent. Loop band around both ankles. Raise knees up toward chest with feet together. Move feet and knees apart.

HOLD: _____ second(s) **REPEAT:** _____ time(s) **FREQUENCY:** _____ x/day

SPECIAL PROTOCOLS/NOTES: Do not arch back. Keep abdominal muscles tight throughout exercise.

_____

_____

PATIENT NAME: _____ DATE: _____

THERAPIST NAME: _____

Supine Hip Adduction

PURPOSE: To strengthen hip and inner thigh muscles.

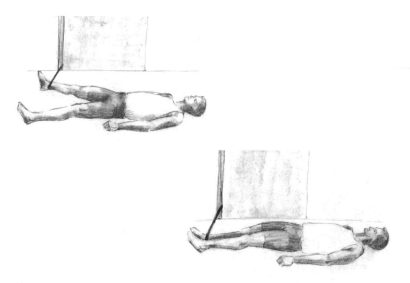

INSTRUCTION: Tie ends of resistive band together and shut knot in door. Loop band around right ankle. Lie on back in neutral position with right side facing door, right ankle close to door, and feet apart. Move right leg in until ankles touch. Repeat with opposite side.

HOLD: _____ second(s) **REPEAT:** _____ time(s) **FREQUENCY:** _____ x/day

SPECIAL PROTOCOLS/NOTES: _____

_____

_____

_____

PATIENT NAME: _____   DATE: _____

THERAPIST NAME: _____

Supine Hip Adduction in Bed

PURPOSE: To strengthen hip and inner thigh muscles.

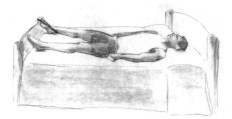

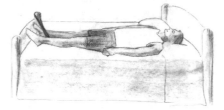

INSTRUCTION: Tie ends of resistive band together. Loop band around bedpost and right ankle. Lie on back in bed in neutral position with feet apart. Move right leg in until ankles touch. Repeat with opposite side.

HOLD: _____ second(s) **REPEAT:** _____ time(s) **FREQUENCY:** _____ x/day

SPECIAL PROTOCOLS/NOTES: _____

_____

_____

_____

PATIENT NAME: _____ DATE: _____

THERAPIST NAME: _____

Supine Hip Adduction/Abduction with Small Ball

PURPOSE: To strengthen inner and outer thigh muscles.

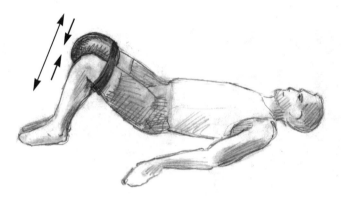

INSTRUCTION: Tie ends of resistive band together. Loop band around both thighs and place small ball between knees. Lie on back in neutral position with knees bent and heels together. Press knees into ball. Hold _____ second(s). Move knees apart without moving feet.

REPEAT: _____ time(s)   **FREQUENCY:** _____ x/day

SPECIAL PROTOCOLS/NOTES: _____
_____
_____
_____

PATIENT NAME: _____ DATE: _____
THERAPIST NAME: _____

Supine Hip Adduction/Abduction with Small Ball While Doing Kegel Exercise

PURPOSE: To strengthen inner and outer thigh and pelvic floor muscles.

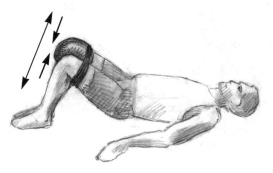

INSTRUCTION: Tie ends of resistive band together. Loop band around both thighs and place small ball between knees. Lie on back in neutral position with knees bent. Gently press knees into ball while tightening pelvic floor muscles. Hold _____ seconds. Slowly relax pelvic floor muscles and knees. Move knees apart without moving feet.

REPEAT: _____ time(s)   **FREQUENCY:** _____ x/day

SPECIAL PROTOCOLS/NOTES: _____
_____
_____
_____

PATIENT NAME: _____ DATE: _____
THERAPIST NAME: _____

Supine Hip Internal Rotation in Bed

PURPOSE: To strengthen buttock and hip muscles.

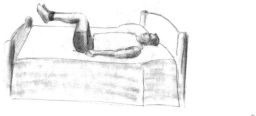

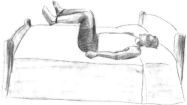

INSTRUCTION: Tie ends of resistive band together. Lie on back in bed in neutral position. Loop band around both ankles. Bend knees and hips to 90°. Move feet apart without moving knees.

HOLD: _____ second(s) **REPEAT:** _____ time(s) **FREQUENCY:** _____ x/day

SPECIAL PROTOCOLS/NOTES: Keep abdominal muscles tight throughout exercise. _____
_____
_____

PATIENT NAME: _____   DATE: _____

THERAPIST NAME: _____

Supine Hip External Rotation in Bed

PURPOSE: To strengthen buttock and hip muscles.

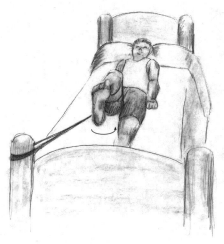

INSTRUCTION: Tie ends of resistive band together. Lie on back in bed in neutral position. Loop band around bedpost and right ankle. Bend right knee and hip to 90°. Move foot, without moving knee, in toward left leg. Repeat with opposite side.

HOLD: _____ second(s) **REPEAT:** _____ time(s) **FREQUENCY:** _____ x/day

SPECIAL PROTOCOLS/NOTES: Keep abdominal muscles tight throughout exercise.

_____

_____

PATIENT NAME: _____ DATE: _____

THERAPIST NAME: _____

Supine on Elbows Leg Press

PURPOSE: To strengthen abdominal, leg, and thigh muscles.

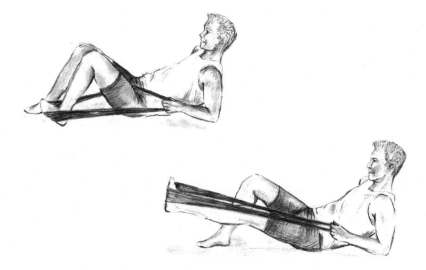

INSTRUCTION: Tie ends of resistive band together. Lie on back in neutral position supported on elbows. Bend both knees. Loop band underneath left forefoot and straighten knee. Repeat with opposite side.

HOLD: _____ second(s) **REPEAT:** _____ time(s) **FREQUENCY:** _____ x/day

SPECIAL PROTOCOLS/NOTES: Keep heel on floor. _____

_____

_____

_____

PATIENT NAME: _____ DATE: _____

THERAPIST NAME: _____

Supine Leg Press in Bed

PURPOSE: To strengthen abdominal, leg, and thigh muscles.

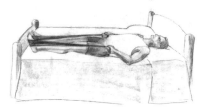

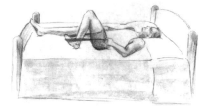

INSTRUCTION: Lie on back in bed in neutral position. Wrap ends of resistive band around each hand. Bend right knee. Loop band underneath right foot. Straighten right leg. Repeat with opposite side.

HOLD: _____ second(s) **REPEAT:** _____ time(s) **FREQUENCY:** _____ x/day

SPECIAL PROTOCOLS/NOTES: _____

_____

_____

_____

PATIENT NAME: _____ DATE: _____

THERAPIST NAME: _____

Supine Double Leg Press

PURPOSE: To strengthen abdominal, leg, and thigh muscles.

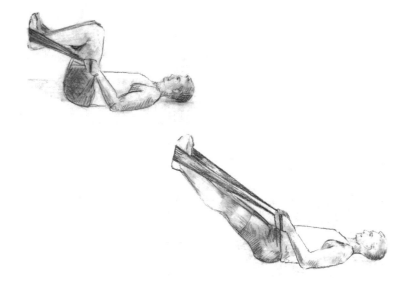

INSTRUCTION: Lie on back in neutral position with knees bent. Bend both knees toward chest. Wrap ends of resistive band around each hand. Loop band underneath both feet. Push both feet out at an angle.

HOLD: _____ second(s) **REPEAT:** _____ time(s) **FREQUENCY:** _____ x/day

SPECIAL PROTOCOLS/NOTES: Do not arch back. Keep abdominal muscles tight throughout exercise. Do not hold breath.

_____

_____

PATIENT NAME: _____ DATE: _____

THERAPIST NAME: _____

Supine Straight Leg Raise

PURPOSE: To strengthen hip, thigh, and leg muscles.

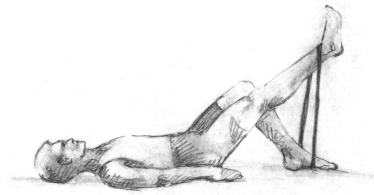

INSTRUCTION: Tie ends of resistive band together. Lie on back in neutral position with both knees bent. Loop band underneath left forefoot and around right ankle. Straighten right leg. Raise right leg. Repeat with opposite side.

HOLD: _____ second(s) **REPEAT:** _____ time(s) **FREQUENCY:** _____ x/day

SPECIAL PROTOCOLS/NOTES: Do not arch back. Keep abdominal muscles tight throughout exercise.

_____

_____

_____

PATIENT NAME: _____ DATE: _____

THERAPIST NAME: _____

Supine Straight Leg Raise with Ball Under Foot

PURPOSE: To strengthen hip, thigh, and leg muscles. To improve balance reactions and coordination.

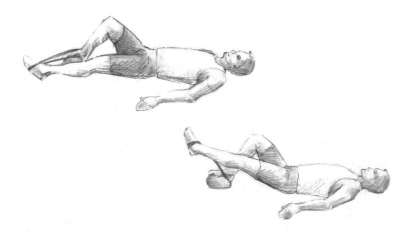

INSTRUCTION: Tie ends of resistive band together. Lie on back in neutral position with both knees bent. Loop band and small ball underneath right forefoot. Straighten left leg and loop band around left ankle. Raise left leg. Repeat with opposite side.

HOLD: _____ second(s) **REPEAT:** _____ time(s) **FREQUENCY:** _____ x/day

SPECIAL PROTOCOLS/NOTES: Do not arch back. Keep abdominal muscles tight throughout exercise. _____

_____

_____

_____

PATIENT NAME: _____ DATE: _____

THERAPIST NAME: _____

Supine Short Arc Quad in Bed

PURPOSE: To strengthen front of thigh muscles.

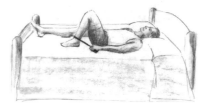

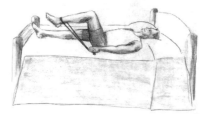

INSTRUCTION: Lie on back in neutral position. Wrap ends of resistive band around each hand. Bend left knee. Loop band around left ankle. Slightly straighten left knee. Repeat with opposite side.

HOLD: _____ second(s) **REPEAT:** _____ time(s) **FREQUENCY:** _____ x/day

SPECIAL PROTOCOLS/NOTES: _____

_____

_____

_____

PATIENT NAME: _____ DATE: _____

THERAPIST NAME: _____

Supine Unilateral Knee Extension

PURPOSE: To strengthen abdominal, leg, and thigh muscles.

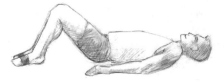

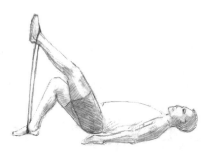

INSTRUCTION: Tie ends of resistive band together. Lie on back in neutral position. Bend both knees. Loop band around both feet. Straighten left knee. Repeat with opposite side.

HOLD: _____ second(s) **REPEAT:** _____ time(s) **FREQUENCY:** _____ x/day

SPECIAL PROTOCOLS/NOTES: _____

_____

_____

_____

PATIENT NAME: _____ DATE: _____

THERAPIST NAME: _____

Supine Bilateral Knee Extension

PURPOSE: To strengthen abdominal, leg, and thigh muscles.

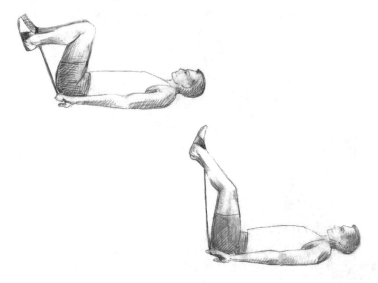

INSTRUCTION: Lie on back in neutral position. Wrap ends of resistive band around each hand. Bend both knees. Loop band around both feet. Place hands underneath buttocks. Straighten knees.

HOLD: _____ second(s) **REPEAT:** _____ time(s) **FREQUENCY:** _____ x/day

SPECIAL PROTOCOLS/NOTES: _____
_____
_____
_____

PATIENT NAME: _____ DATE: _____
THERAPIST NAME: _____

Supine Ankle Plantarflexion

PURPOSE: To strengthen calf muscles.

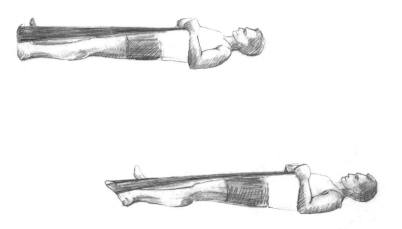

INSTRUCTION: Tie ends of resistive band together and hold knot in both hands. Lie on back. Loop band around left forefoot. Push toes of left foot down. Repeat with opposite side.

HOLD: _____ second(s) **REPEAT:** _____ time(s) **FREQUENCY:** _____ x/day

SPECIAL PROTOCOLS/NOTES: _____

_____

_____

_____

PATIENT NAME: _____   DATE: _____

THERAPIST NAME: _____

Supine Ankle Dorsiflexion

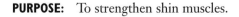

PURPOSE: To strengthen shin muscles.

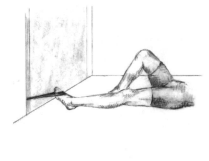
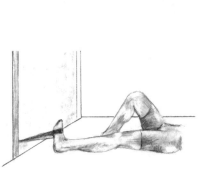

INSTRUCTION: Tie ends of resistive band together and shut knot in door. Lie on back, facing door. Loop band around left forefoot. Pull toes of left foot up toward nose. Repeat with opposite side.

HOLD: _____ second(s) **REPEAT:** _____ time(s) **FREQUENCY:** _____ x/day

SPECIAL PROTOCOLS/NOTES: _____

_____

_____

_____

PATIENT NAME: _____ DATE: _____

THERAPIST NAME: _____

Supine Ankle Inversion

PURPOSE: To strengthen inner ankle muscles.

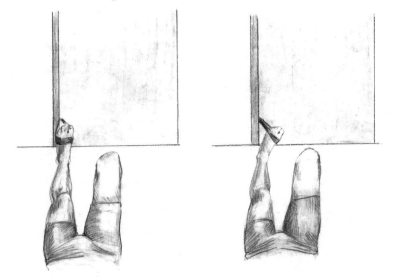

INSTRUCTION: Tie ends of resistive band together and shut knot in door. Lie on back, facing door. Loop band around left forefoot. Move toes of left foot up and in toward right knee. Repeat with opposite side.

HOLD: _____ second(s) **REPEAT:** _____ time(s) **FREQUENCY:** _____ x/day

SPECIAL PROTOCOLS/NOTES: _____
_____
_____
_____

PATIENT NAME: _____ DATE: _____

THERAPIST NAME: _____

Supine Ankle Eversion

PURPOSE: To strengthen outer ankle muscles.

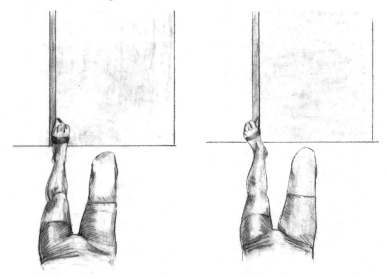

INSTRUCTION: Tie ends of resistive band together and shut knot in door. Lie on back, facing door. Loop band around left forefoot. Move toes of left foot up and out toward outer shin. Repeat with opposite side.

HOLD: _____ second(s) **REPEAT:** _____ time(s) **FREQUENCY:** _____ x/day

SPECIAL PROTOCOLS/NOTES: _____

_____

_____

_____

PATIENT NAME: _____ DATE: _____

THERAPIST NAME: _____

Supine Ankle Eversion II

PURPOSE: To strengthen outer ankle muscles.

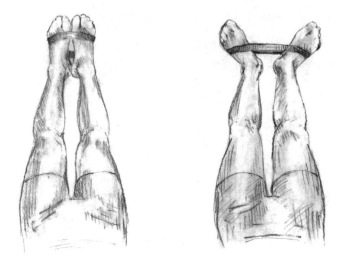

INSTRUCTION: Tie ends of resistive band together. Loop band around both forefeet. Lie on back with legs out straight. Move toes away from each other.

HOLD: _____ second(s) **REPEAT:** _____ time(s) **FREQUENCY:** _____ x/day

SPECIAL PROTOCOLS/NOTES: _____
_____
_____
_____

PATIENT NAME: _____ DATE: _____

THERAPIST NAME: _____

Sport-Specific Exercises

CHAPTER EIGHT

Baseball Throw

PURPOSE: To strengthen arm, shoulder, and wrist muscles.

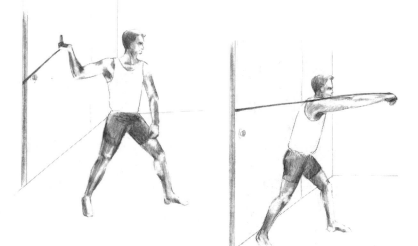

INSTRUCTION: Tie knot in one end of resistive band and shut knot in door. Stand in neutral position with left foot in front of the right, facing away from door. Loop other end of band around right hand. Bend right wrist and elbow back behind head. Rotate hand and shoulder forward as if throwing baseball. Follow through with arm straight, palm down, and transfer weight forward to left leg. Repeat with opposite side.

HOLD: _____ second(s) **REPEAT:** _____ time(s) **FREQUENCY:** _____ x/day

SPECIAL PROTOCOLS/NOTES: _____
_____
_____
_____

PATIENT NAME: _____ DATE: _____

THERAPIST NAME: _____

Basketball Free Throw

PURPOSE: To strengthen arm, forearm, and wrist muscles.

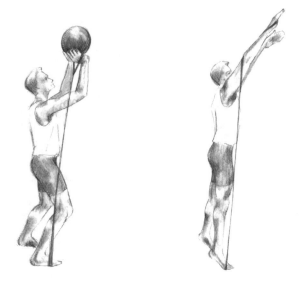

INSTRUCTION: Stand in neutral position with feet shoulder-width apart and right foot slightly in front of the left. Loop resistive band around right hand and step on other end of band with right foot. Bend wrist back and place ball in hand. Bend both knees. Shoot basketball into hoop by flicking wrist forward, extending arms, and knees and raising up onto toes. Repeat with opposite side.

HOLD: _____ second(s) **REPEAT:** _____ time(s) **FREQUENCY:** _____ x/day

SPECIAL PROTOCOLS/NOTES: _____

_____

_____

_____

PATIENT NAME: _____ DATE: _____

THERAPIST NAME: _____

Bench Press on Ball

PURPOSE: To strengthen arm, leg, and back muscles.

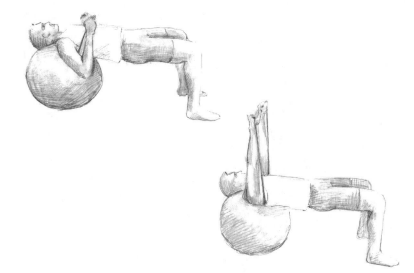

INSTRUCTION: Sit on ball. Loop resistive band behind back and grasp ends of band in both hands. Walk legs out away from ball so head and shoulders rest on ball. Bend elbows as shown. Raise both arms up toward ceiling.

HOLD: _____ second(s) **REPEAT:** _____ time(s) **FREQUENCY:** _____ x/day

SPECIAL PROTOCOLS/NOTES: _____

_____

_____

_____

PATIENT NAME: _____ DATE: _____

THERAPIST NAME: _____

Boxing Jab

PURPOSE: To strengthen arm, chest, and shoulder muscles.

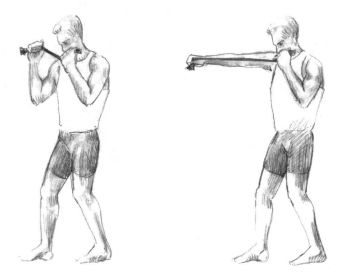

INSTRUCTION: Stand with right foot in front of left foot. Bend both elbows. Grasp ends of resistive band with both hands. Raise both hands to shoulder height and position right hand in front of left hand. Quickly punch right hand out and rotate palm down.

HOLD: _____ second(s) **REPEAT:** _____ time(s) **FREQUENCY:** _____ x/day

SPECIAL PROTOCOLS/NOTES: _____

_____

_____

_____

PATIENT NAME: _____ DATE: _____

THERAPIST NAME: _____

Boxing Reverse Arm Punch

PURPOSE: To strengthen arm, chest, and shoulder muscles.

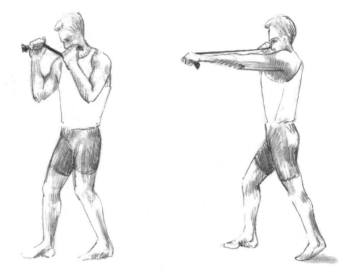

INSTRUCTION: Stand with right foot in front of left foot. Bend both elbows. Grasp ends of resistive band with both hands. Raise hands to shoulder height and position right hand in front of left hand. Quickly punch left hand out and rotate palm down as body weight shifts forward over right foot and left heel raises off floor.

HOLD: _____ second(s) **REPEAT:** _____ time(s) **FREQUENCY:** _____ x/day

SPECIAL PROTOCOLS/NOTES: _____

_____
_____
_____

PATIENT NAME: _____ DATE: _____

THERAPIST NAME: _____

Golf Swing

PURPOSE: To strengthen arm, shoulder, and trunk muscles.

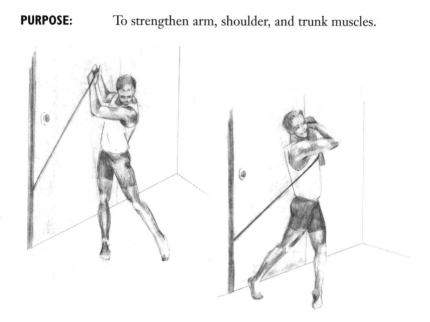

INSTRUCTION: Tie knot in one end of resistive band and shut knot in door at knee height. Wrap other end of band around right hand. Stand with right hip toward door. Raise both hands over right shoulder keeping eyes on golf ball. Follow through with hands as if swinging club. Repeat with opposite side.

HOLD: _____ second(s) **REPEAT:** _____ time(s) **FREQUENCY:** _____ x/day

SPECIAL PROTOCOLS/NOTES: _____

_____

_____

_____

PATIENT NAME: _____ DATE: _____

THERAPIST NAME: _____

Kick Boxing

PURPOSE: To strengthen abdominal, back, hip, leg, and thigh muscles.

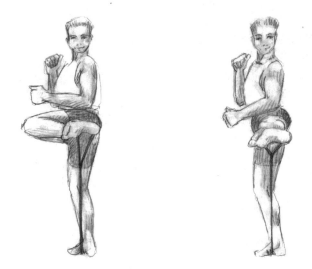

INSTRUCTION: Stand in neutral position. Loop one end of resistive band around left foot and step on other end of band with right foot. Rotate right foot out away from body. Turn head to left. Bend both elbows and raise right hand to shoulder. Bend left knee and raise left leg out away from body. Punch left leg out away from left side of body, keeping left foot parallel to floor. Return to standing neutral position.

HOLD: _____ second(s) **REPEAT:** _____ time(s) **FREQUENCY:** _____ x/day

SPECIAL PROTOCOLS/NOTES: Do not arch back. _____

_____

_____

_____

PATIENT NAME: _____ DATE: _____

THERAPIST NAME: _____

Running

PURPOSE: To strengthen arm, forearm, and shoulder muscles.

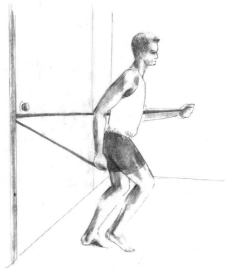

INSTRUCTION: Tie knot in middle of resistive band and shut knot in door at elbow height. Wrap ends of band around each hand. Stand facing away from door. Alternate swinging each arm forward and back while running in place.

HOLD: _____ second(s) **REPEAT:** _____ time(s) **FREQUENCY:** _____ x/day

SPECIAL PROTOCOLS/NOTES: When running, right knee bends and raises as left arm swings forward, and vice versa for opposite side.

_____

_____

PATIENT NAME: _____   DATE: _____

THERAPIST NAME: _____

Shoulder Press

PURPOSE: To strengthen shoulder muscles.

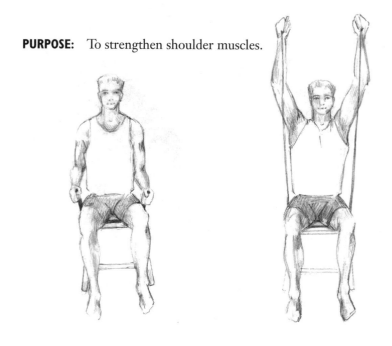

INSTRUCTION: Sit in neutral position. Grasp ends of resistive band with both hands. Loop band under both thighs. Raise both arms straight up toward ceiling.

HOLD: _____ second(s) **REPEAT:** _____ time(s) **FREQUENCY:** _____ x/day

SPECIAL PROTOCOLS/NOTES: _____

_____

_____

_____

PATIENT NAME: _____ DATE: _____

THERAPIST NAME: _____

Skiing — Cross-Country

PURPOSE: To strengthen arm, forearm, and shoulder muscles.

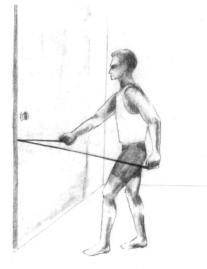

INSTRUCTION: Tie knot in middle of resistive band and shut knot in door at elbow height. Wrap ends of band around each hand. Stand facing door. Place left foot in front of right. Alternate swinging each arm forward and back. Repeat with opposite foot forward.

HOLD: _____ second(s) **REPEAT:** _____ time(s) **FREQUENCY:** _____ x/day

SPECIAL PROTOCOLS/NOTES: _____
_____
_____
_____

PATIENT NAME: _____ DATE: _____
THERAPIST NAME: _____

Soccer Pass Behind Body

PURPOSE: To strengthen foot, thigh, and leg muscles.
To improve balance.

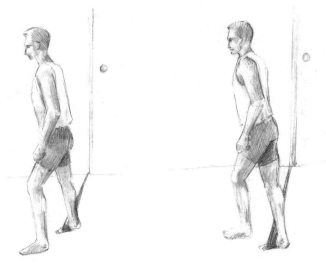

INSTRUCTION: Tie ends of resistive band together and shut knot in bottom of door. Stand with right side toward door. Loop band around right forefoot. Straighten right leg back behind body. Rapidly move right foot back behind left heel, as if passing the ball. Repeat with opposite side.

HOLD: _____ second(s) **REPEAT:** _____ time(s) **FREQUENCY:** _____ x/day

SPECIAL PROTOCOLS/NOTES: _____

_____

_____

_____

PATIENT NAME: _____ DATE: _____

THERAPIST NAME: _____

Soccer Pass in Front of Body

PURPOSE: To strengthen foot, thigh, and leg muscles.
To improve balance.

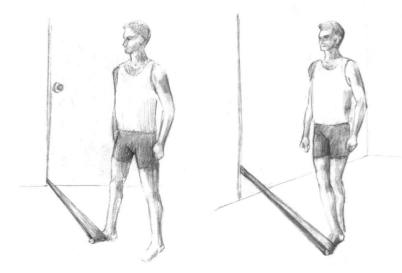

INSTRUCTION: Tie ends of resistive band together and shut knot in bottom of door. Stand with right side toward door and right leg slightly in front of left. Loop band around right forefoot. Rapidly move right foot across left foot, as if passing the ball. Repeat with opposite side.

HOLD: _____ second(s) **REPEAT:** _____ time(s) **FREQUENCY:** _____ x/day

SPECIAL PROTOCOLS/NOTES: _____
_____
_____
_____

PATIENT NAME: _____ DATE: _____

THERAPIST NAME: _____

Speed Skating

PURPOSE: To strengthen leg and thigh muscles.

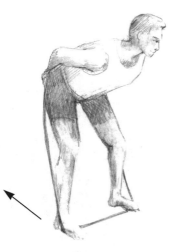

INSTRUCTION: Stand with right foot in front of left. Wrap ends of resistive band around each hand. Loop band under both feet. Bend at waist with both hands behind back. Push and straighten right leg back behind body. Return to starting position. Repeat with left leg.

HOLD: _____ second(s) **REPEAT:** _____ time(s) **FREQUENCY:** _____ x/day

SPECIAL PROTOCOLS/NOTES: _____

_____

_____

_____

PATIENT NAME: _____ DATE: _____

THERAPIST NAME: _____

Swimming—Backstroke on Ball

PURPOSE: To strengthen arm, back, leg, and shoulder muscles.

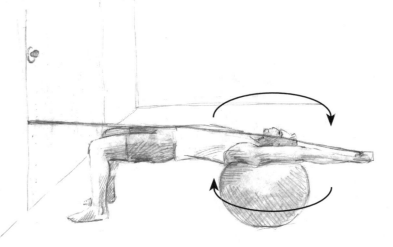

INSTRUCTION: Tie knot in one end of resistive band and shut knot in door at knee height. Grasp ends of band in both hands. Sit on ball, facing door. Walk legs out away from ball so head and shoulders rest on ball. Straighten one arm, raise overhead, and backstroke. Alternate backstroking with each arm.

HOLD: _____ second(s) **REPEAT:** _____ time(s) **FREQUENCY:** _____ x/day

SPECIAL PROTOCOLS/NOTES: _____

_____

_____

_____

PATIENT NAME: _____ DATE: _____

THERAPIST NAME: _____

Swimming — Freestyle on Ball

PURPOSE: To strengthen arm, back, leg, neck, and shoulder muscles.

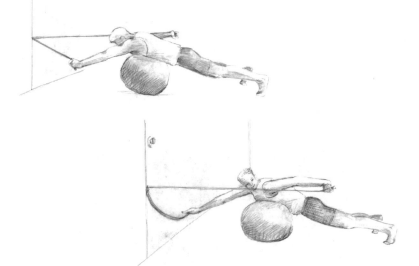

INSTRUCTION: Tie knot in middle of resistive band and shut knot in door at knee height. Grasp ends of band in both hands. Lie facing door with abdomen on ball and legs out straight. Raise right arm overhead and lower left arm down by side of body. Begin freestyle swimming, alternating arms and rotating head when appropriate.

HOLD: _____ second(s) **REPEAT:** _____ time(s) **FREQUENCY:** _____ x/day

SPECIAL PROTOCOLS/NOTES: _____
_____
_____
_____

PATIENT NAME: _____ DATE: _____

THERAPIST NAME: _____

Tennis — Backhand

PURPOSE: To strengthen wrist, arm, forearm, and shoulder muscles.

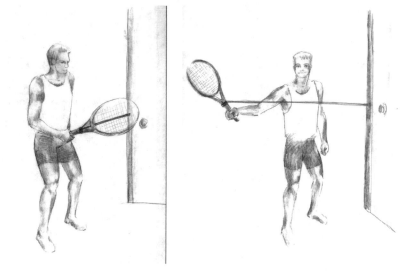

INSTRUCTION: Tie knot in one end of resistive band and shut knot in door at elbow height. Wrap other end of band around tennis racquet. Stand with left hip toward door and right hand holding racquet with thumb toward ceiling. Swing racquet up, out, and away in backhand position. Repeat with opposite side.

HOLD: _____ second(s) **REPEAT:** _____ time(s) **FREQUENCY:** _____ x/day

SPECIAL PROTOCOLS/NOTES: _____

_____

_____

_____

PATIENT NAME: _____ DATE: _____

THERAPIST NAME: _____

Tennis — Forehand

PURPOSE: To strengthen arm, forearm, shoulder, and wrist muscles.

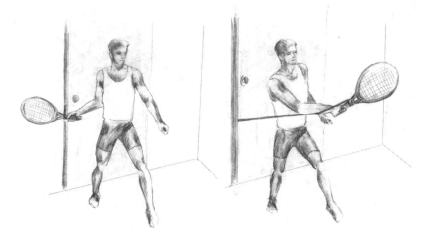

INSTRUCTION: Tie knot in one end of resistive band and shut knot in door at elbow height. Wrap other end of band around tennis racquet. Stand with left foot in front of the right and right hand, thumb up, holding racquet to side and back of body. Swing racquet across body in a forehand swing. Follow through with racquet coming up and over left shoulder while taking a step forward with right foot. Repeat with opposite side.

HOLD: _____ second(s) **REPEAT:** _____ time(s) **FREQUENCY:** _____ x/day

SPECIAL PROTOCOLS/NOTES: _____

_____

_____

_____

PATIENT NAME: _____ DATE: _____

THERAPIST NAME: _____

Volleyball — Set

PURPOSE: To strengthen arm, shoulder, and wrist muscles.

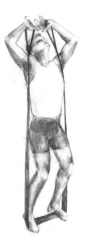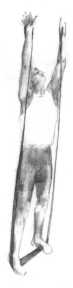

INSTRUCTION: Stand in neutral position with feet shoulder-width apart. Wrap ends of band around each hand. Loop band under both feet. Bend both knees and raise hands up above head forming a triangle between index fingers and thumbs. Straighten both arms overhead turning thumbs in as if setting ball. Return to starting position.

HOLD: _____ second(s) **REPEAT:** _____ time(s) **FREQUENCY:** _____ x/day

SPECIAL PROTOCOLS/NOTES: _____

_____

_____

_____

PATIENT NAME: _____ DATE: _____

THERAPIST NAME: _____

Volleyball — Spike

PURPOSE: To strengthen arm, shoulder, and wrist muscles.

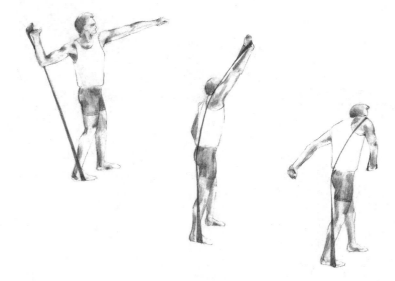

INSTRUCTION: Stand in neutral position with left foot in front of the right. Loop resistive band under right foot and wrap other end of band around right hand. Bend right elbow, raise to shoulder height and rotate right side of trunk back. Straighten right arm overhead as if hitting ball. Follow through with arm, rotating trunk to left and lowering arm. Return to starting position. Repeat with opposite side.

HOLD: _____ second(s) **REPEAT:** _____ time(s) **FREQUENCY:** _____ x/day

SPECIAL PROTOCOLS/NOTES: _____
_____
_____
_____

PATIENT NAME: _____ DATE: _____

THERAPIST NAME: _____

Weight Lifting Back Squat

PURPOSE: To strengthen buttock, leg, and shoulder muscles.

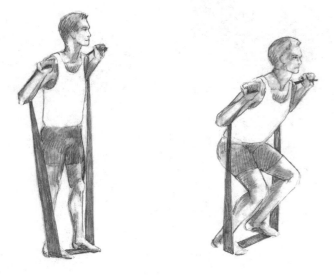

INSTRUCTION: Stand in neutral position with feet shoulder-width apart. Wrap ends of resistive band around each hand. Loop band under both feet. Raise both hands up to shoulders with knuckles facing forward. Bend knees.

HOLD: _____ second(s) **REPEAT:** _____ time(s) **FREQUENCY:** _____ x/day

SPECIAL PROTOCOLS/NOTES: _____
_____
_____
_____

PATIENT NAME: _____ DATE: _____

THERAPIST NAME: _____

Resistive Band and Resistive Band Strip Hand Exercises

CHAPTER NINE

Thumb Flexion/Opposition

PURPOSE: To strengthen palm and thumb muscles.

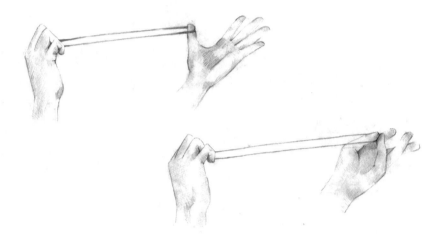

INSTRUCTION: Loop resistive band strip around left thumb. Hold other end of band with right hand. Pull band across left palm and touch pinky tip. Repeat with right hand.

HOLD: _____ second(s) **REPEAT:** _____ time(s) **FREQUENCY:** _____ x/day

SPECIAL PROTOCOLS/NOTES: _____
_____
_____
_____

PATIENT NAME: _____ DATE: _____

THERAPIST NAME: _____

Thumb Extension

PURPOSE: To strengthen thumb muscles.

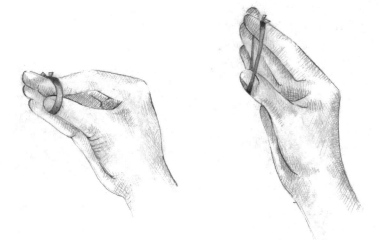

INSTRUCTION: Loop resistive band strip around right thumb and base of index finger. Move thumb out away from index finger. Repeat with left thumb.

HOLD: _____ second(s) **REPEAT:** _____ time(s) **FREQUENCY:** _____ x/day

SPECIAL PROTOCOLS/NOTES: _____
_____
_____
_____

PATIENT NAME: _____ DATE: _____

THERAPIST NAME: _____

Thumb Abduction

PURPOSE: To strengthen thumb muscles.

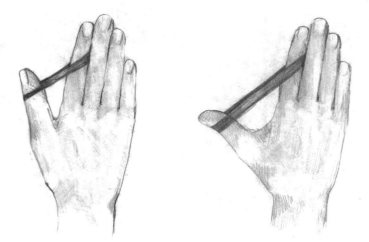

INSTRUCTION: Loop resistive band strip around right thumb and index
finger. Move thumb out away from index finger. Repeat
with left thumb.

HOLD: _____ second(s) **REPEAT:** _____ time(s) **FREQUENCY:** _____ x/day

SPECIAL PROTOCOLS/NOTES: _____

_____

_____

_____

PATIENT NAME: _____   DATE: _____

THERAPIST NAME: _____

Thumb Adduction

PURPOSE: To strengthen inner thumb muscles.

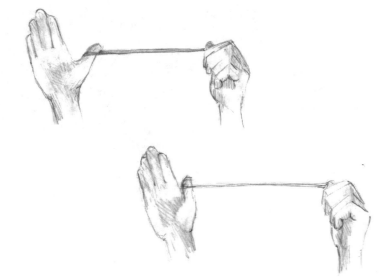

INSTRUCTION: Loop resistive band strip around right thumb and hold
other end of band with left hand. Move right thumb out
away from index finger. Pull band in toward index finger. Repeat with left thumb.

HOLD: _____ second(s) **REPEAT:** _____ time(s) **FREQUENCY:** _____ x/day

SPECIAL PROTOCOLS/NOTES: _____

_____

_____

_____

PATIENT NAME: _____ DATE: _____

THERAPIST NAME: _____

Individual Finger Flexion

PURPOSE: To strengthen finger muscles.

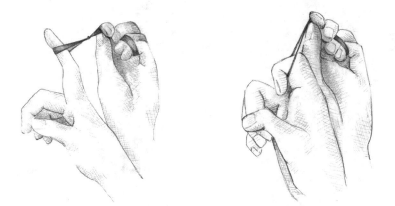

INSTRUCTION: Loop resistive band strip around one finger on right hand and hold other end of band with left hand. Straighten finger. Bend fingertip toward palm. Repeat with each finger on right hand. Repeat with left hand.

HOLD: _____ second(s) **REPEAT:** _____ time(s) **FREQUENCY:** _____ x/day

SPECIAL PROTOCOLS/NOTES: _____
_____
_____
_____

PATIENT NAME: _____ DATE: _____

THERAPIST NAME: _____

Four Finger Flexion

PURPOSE: To strengthen finger and palm muscles.

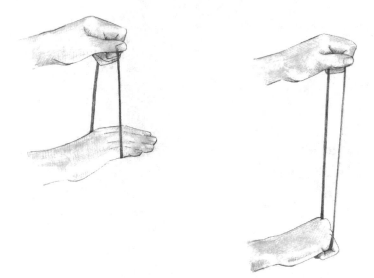

INSTRUCTION: Loop resistive band strip around right four fingers and hold other end of band with left. Straighten fingers on right hand. Bend fingertips toward palm as with making a fist. Repeat with left hand.

HOLD: _____ second(s) **REPEAT:** _____ time(s) **FREQUENCY:** _____ x/day

SPECIAL PROTOCOLS/NOTES: _____

_____

_____

_____

PATIENT NAME: _____ DATE: _____

THERAPIST NAME: _____

Individual Finger Extension

PURPOSE: To strengthen finger muscles.

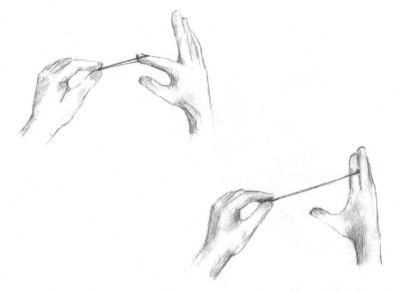

INSTRUCTION: Loop resistive band strip around one finger on right hand and hold other end of band with left hand. Bend fingertip toward palm. Straighten finger. Repeat with each finger on right hand. Repeat with left hand.

HOLD: _____ second(s) **REPEAT:** _____ time(s) **FREQUENCY:** _____ x/day

SPECIAL PROTOCOLS/NOTES: _____
_____
_____
_____

PATIENT NAME: _____ DATE: _____

THERAPIST NAME: _____

Four Finger Extension

PURPOSE: To strengthen finger muscles.

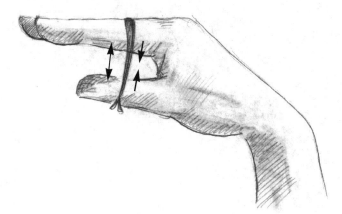

INSTRUCTION: Loop resistive band strip around base of fingers and thumb on right hand. Straighten fingers. Squeeze fingers and thumb together. Raise fingers toward ceiling, keeping fingers straight. Repeat with left hand.

HOLD: _____ second(s) **REPEAT:** _____ time(s) **FREQUENCY:** _____ x/day

SPECIAL PROTOCOLS/NOTES: _____
_____
_____
_____

PATIENT NAME: _____ DATE: _____
THERAPIST NAME: _____

Triangular Finger Extension

PURPOSE: To strengthen finger muscles.

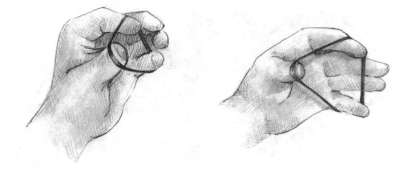

INSTRUCTION: Loop resistive band strip around tip of thumb, index, and pinky fingers of right hand. Squeeze fingers and thumb together. Raise fingers toward ceiling. Repeat exercise with thumb, middle, and pinky fingers; and with thumb, ring, and pinky fingers of right hand. Repeat with left hand.

HOLD: _____ second(s) **REPEAT:** _____ time(s) **FREQUENCY:** _____ x/day

SPECIAL PROTOCOLS/NOTES: _____
_____
_____
_____

PATIENT NAME: _____ DATE: _____

THERAPIST NAME: _____

Finger Adduction

PURPOSE: To strengthen inner finger muscles.

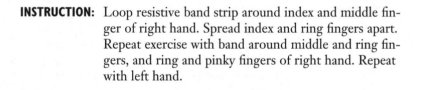

INSTRUCTION: Loop resistive band strip around index and middle finger of right hand. Spread index and ring fingers apart. Repeat exercise with band around middle and ring fingers, and ring and pinky fingers of right hand. Repeat with left hand.

HOLD: _____ second(s) **REPEAT:** _____ time(s) **FREQUENCY:** _____ x/day

SPECIAL PROTOCOLS/NOTES: _____
_____
_____
_____

PATIENT NAME: _____ DATE: _____

THERAPIST NAME: _____

Four Finger Adduction

PURPOSE: To strengthen inner finger muscles.

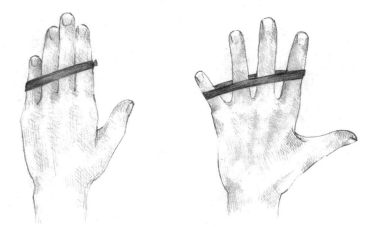

INSTRUCTION: Loop resistive band strip around all four fingers of right hand. Spread fingers apart. Repeat with left hand.

HOLD: _____ second(s) **REPEAT:** _____ time(s) **FREQUENCY:** _____ x/day

SPECIAL PROTOCOLS/NOTES: _____
_____
_____
_____

PATIENT NAME: _____ DATE: _____

THERAPIST NAME: _____

Wrist Flexion/Extension Twist

PURPOSE: To strengthen wrist muscles.

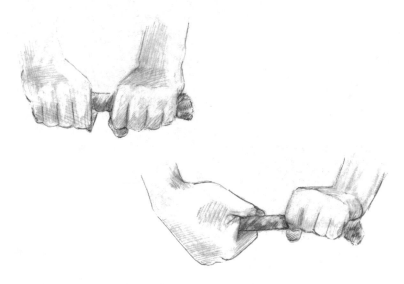

INSTRUCTION: Sit in neutral position. Fold four feet of resistive band back and forth, eight times. Bend both elbows with palms down and grasp band. Bend one wrist forward and opposite wrist backward, as if wringing out a wet towel. Repeat in opposite direction.

HOLD: _____ second(s) **REPEAT:** _____ time(s) **FREQUENCY:** _____ x/day

SPECIAL PROTOCOLS/NOTES: Do not lift forearms. _____

_____

_____

_____

PATIENT NAME: _____ DATE: _____

THERAPIST NAME: _____

Wrist Radial Deviation
in Pronation

PURPOSE: To strengthen wrist muscles.

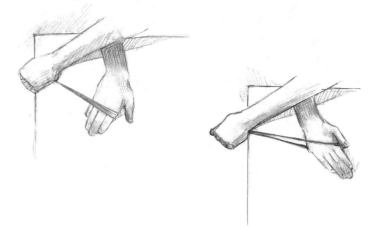

INSTRUCTION: Sit in neutral position. Loop resistive band around right hand and place hand on table with palm down. Hold other end of band in left hand and cross left hand over right. Move right hand toward and away from left hand. Repeat with left hand.

HOLD: _____ second(s) **REPEAT:** _____ time(s) **FREQUENCY:** _____ x/day

SPECIAL PROTOCOLS/NOTES: Do not move forearm. _____

_____

_____

_____

PATIENT NAME: _____ DATE: _____

THERAPIST NAME: _____

Wrist Ulnar Deviation
in Pronation

PURPOSE: To strengthen wrist muscles.

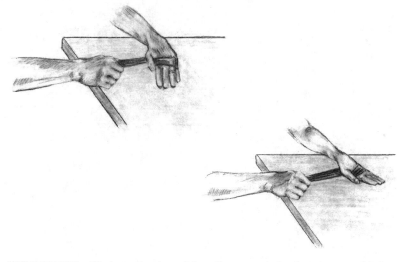

INSTRUCTION: Sit in neutral position. Loop resistive band around left hand and place hand on table with palm down. Move hand toward body and then away from body. Repeat with right hand.

HOLD: _____ second(s) **REPEAT:** _____ time(s) **FREQUENCY:** _____ x/day

SPECIAL PROTOCOLS/NOTES: <u>Do not move forearm.</u>

_____

_____

_____

PATIENT NAME: _____ DATE: _____

THERAPIST NAME: _____

Wrist Pronation

PURPOSE: To strengthen forearm and wrist muscles.

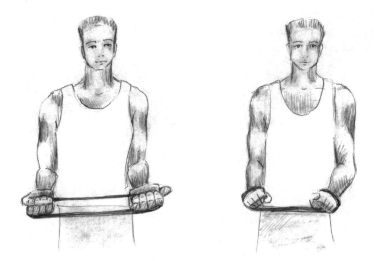

INSTRUCTION: Stand in neutral position with feet shoulder-width apart. Loop resistive band around both hands. Grasp top of loop with palms up. Rotate hands so palms face down.

HOLD: _____ second(s) **REPEAT:** _____ time(s) **FREQUENCY:** _____ x/day

SPECIAL PROTOCOLS/NOTES: Shoulders should not move during exercise.

_____

_____

_____

PATIENT NAME: _____ DATE: _____

THERAPIST NAME: _____

Wrist Supination

PURPOSE: To strengthen forearm and wrist muscles.

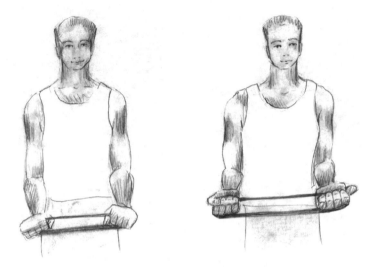

INSTRUCTION: Stand in neutral position with feet shoulder-width apart. Loop resistive band around both hands. Grasp top of loop with palms down. Rotate hands so palms face up.

HOLD: _____ second(s) **REPEAT:** _____ time(s) **FREQUENCY:** _____ x/day

SPECIAL PROTOCOLS/NOTES: Shoulders should not move during exercise.
_____
_____
_____

PATIENT NAME: _____   DATE: _____

THERAPIST NAME: _____

CHAPTER TEN

Resistive Putty

CHAPTER TEN

RESISTIVE PUTTY EXERCISES

HAND/UPPER EXTREMITIES

Tip Pinch

PURPOSE: To strengthen pinch muscles between thumb and index finger.

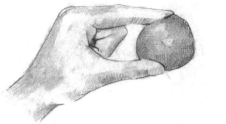

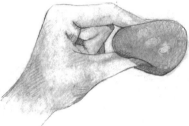

INSTRUCTION: Place putty ball between thumb and index finger of right hand. Squeeze ball. Repeat with left hand.

HOLD: _____ second(s) **REPEAT:** _____ time(s) **FREQUENCY:** _____ x/day

SPECIAL PROTOCOLS/NOTES: _____
_____
_____
_____

PATIENT NAME: _____ DATE: _____
THERAPIST NAME: _____

Three Jaw Grasp

PURPOSE: To strengthen palm and thumb muscles.

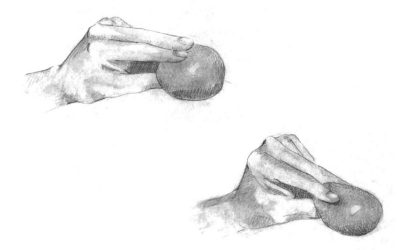

INSTRUCTION: Place putty ball between thumb, index, and middle finger of right hand. Squeeze ball. Repeat with left hand.

HOLD: _____ second(s) **REPEAT:** _____ time(s) **FREQUENCY:** _____ x/day

SPECIAL PROTOCOLS/NOTES: _____
_____
_____
_____

PATIENT NAME: _____ DATE: _____

THERAPIST NAME: _____

Lateral Pinch

PURPOSE: To strengthen pinch muscles between thumb and index finger.

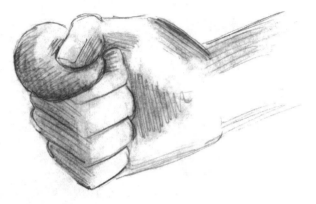

INSTRUCTION: Place putty ball between thumb and index finger of right hand. Squeeze ball. Repeat with left hand.

HOLD: _____ second(s) **REPEAT:** _____ time(s) **FREQUENCY:** _____ x/day

SPECIAL PROTOCOLS/NOTES: _____
_____
_____
_____

PATIENT NAME: _____ DATE: _____

THERAPIST NAME: _____

Pinch and Pull

PURPOSE: To strengthen finger and thumb muscles.

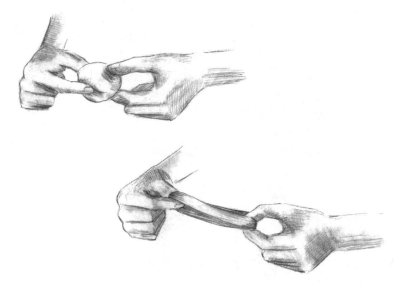

INSTRUCTION: Place putty ball in right hand. Pinch putty with thumb and index finger and pull. Repeat with thumb and middle finger, thumb and ring finger, and thumb and pinky finger of the right hand. Repeat with left hand.

HOLD: _____ second(s) **REPEAT:** _____ time(s) **FREQUENCY:** _____ x/day

SPECIAL PROTOCOLS/NOTES: _____
_____
_____
_____

PATIENT NAME: _____ DATE: _____

THERAPIST NAME: _____

Horizontal Abduction Pull

PURPOSE: To strengthen finger and wrist muscles.

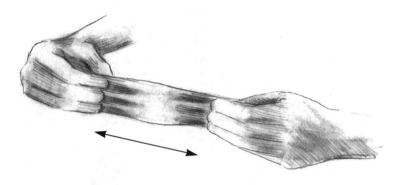

INSTRUCTION: Place putty ball in both hands. Pinch each end of putty with thumb and fingers. Pull hands apart as if pulling taffy.

HOLD: _____ second(s) **REPEAT:** _____ time(s) **FREQUENCY:** _____ x/day

SPECIAL PROTOCOLS/NOTES: _____

_____

_____

_____

PATIENT NAME: _____ DATE: _____

THERAPIST NAME: _____

Putty Ball Squeeze with Hand

PURPOSE: To strengthen flexor muscles in hand.

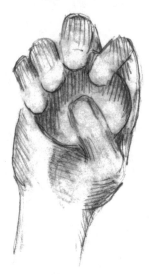

INSTRUCTION: Place putty ball in right hand. Squeeze ball with fingers and thumb. Repeat with left hand.

HOLD: _____ second(s) **REPEAT:** _____ time(s) **FREQUENCY:** _____ x/day

SPECIAL PROTOCOLS/NOTES: _____
_____
_____
_____

PATIENT NAME: _____ DATE: _____
THERAPIST NAME: _____

Thumb Flexion

PURPOSE: To strengthen thumb muscles.

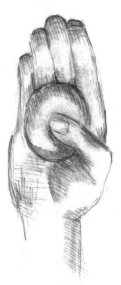

INSTRUCTION: Place putty ball in right hand. Press thumb toward pinky. Repeat with left hand.

HOLD: _____ second(s) **REPEAT:** _____ time(s) **FREQUENCY:** _____ x/day

SPECIAL PROTOCOLS/NOTES: _____

_____

_____

_____

PATIENT NAME: _____ DATE: _____

THERAPIST NAME: _____

Thumb Extension

PURPOSE: To strengthen back side of thumb.

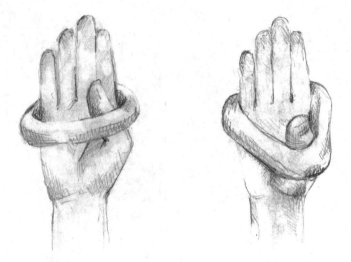

INSTRUCTION: Place a loop of putty around base of fingers and thumb of right hand with thumb touching pinky. Move thumb away from pinky and palm. Repeat with left hand.

HOLD: _____ second(s) **REPEAT:** _____ time(s) **FREQUENCY:** _____ x/day

SPECIAL PROTOCOLS/NOTES: _____

_____

_____

_____

PATIENT NAME: _____ DATE: _____

THERAPIST NAME: _____

Thumb Extension II

PURPOSE: To strengthen thumb muscles.

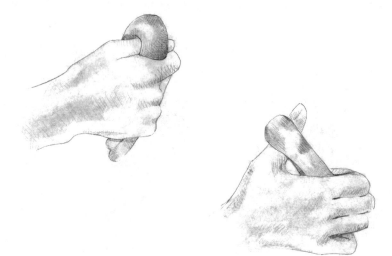

INSTRUCTION: Loop resistive putty around thumb of right hand and hold ends of putty with fingers. Straighten and lift thumb up, as in "thumbs up." Repeat with left hand.

HOLD: _____ second(s) **REPEAT:** _____ time(s) **FREQUENCY:** _____ x/day

SPECIAL PROTOCOLS/NOTES: _____

_____

_____

_____

PATIENT NAME: _____ DATE: _____

THERAPIST NAME: _____

Thumb Flexion/Extension with Putty Cylinder

PURPOSE: To strengthen thumb muscles and improve range of motion.

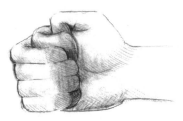

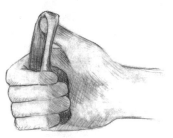

INSTRUCTION: Roll putty into cylindrical shape and place in right hand. Press thumb into putty. Straighten thumb and lift up, as in "thumbs up." Repeat with left hand.

HOLD: _____ second(s) **REPEAT:** _____ time(s) **FREQUENCY:** _____ x/day

SPECIAL PROTOCOLS/NOTES: _____

_____

_____

_____

PATIENT NAME: _____ DATE: _____

THERAPIST NAME: _____

Thumb Extension/
Flexion/Opposition

PURPOSE: To strengthen thumb muscles and increase range of motion.

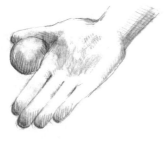
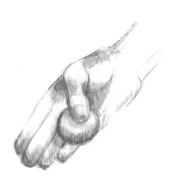

INSTRUCTION: Place putty ball on inside of right thumb. Roll ball toward pinky finger. Return to starting position. Repeat with left hand.

HOLD: _____ second(s) **REPEAT:** _____ time(s) **FREQUENCY:** _____ x/day

SPECIAL PROTOCOLS/NOTES: _____
_____
_____
_____

PATIENT NAME: _____ DATE: _____

THERAPIST NAME: _____

Radial Thumb Abduction

PURPOSE: To strengthen outer thumb muscles.

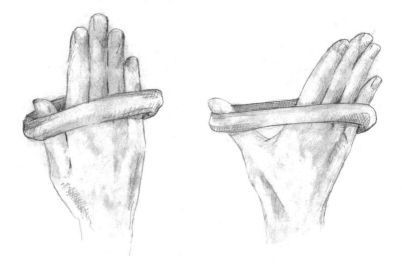

INSTRUCTION: Loop putty around base of fingers and thumb of right hand. Move thumb away from index finger. Repeat with left hand.

HOLD: _____ second(s) **REPEAT:** _____ time(s) **FREQUENCY:** _____ x/day

SPECIAL PROTOCOLS/NOTES: _____
_____
_____
_____

PATIENT NAME: _____ DATE: _____

THERAPIST NAME: _____

Radial Thumb Abduction with Palm Down

PURPOSE: To improve range of motion, strength, and coordination in thumb.

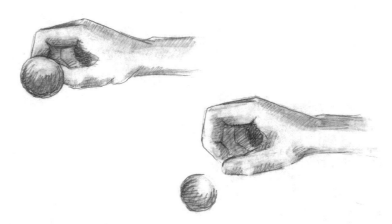

INSTRUCTION: Place right hand on table, palm down. Place ball of putty in front of thumb. Flick ball with thumb. Repeat with left hand.

HOLD: _____ second(s) **REPEAT:** _____ time(s) **FREQUENCY:** _____ x/day

SPECIAL PROTOCOLS/NOTES: _____

_____

_____

_____

PATIENT NAME: _____ DATE: _____

THERAPIST NAME: _____

Radial Thumb Flick

PURPOSE: To strengthen thumb muscles and increase range of motion and coordination.

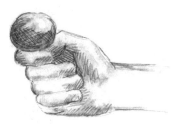
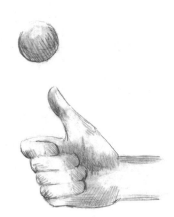

INSTRUCTION: Bend fingers into palm of right hand. Place ball on top of thumb. Flick ball upward with thumb. Repeat with left hand.

HOLD: _____ second(s) **REPEAT:** _____ time(s) **FREQUENCY:** _____ x/day

SPECIAL PROTOCOLS/NOTES: _____
_____
_____
_____

PATIENT NAME: _____ DATE: _____

THERAPIST NAME: _____

Thumb Adduction

PURPOSE: To strengthen thumb muscles.

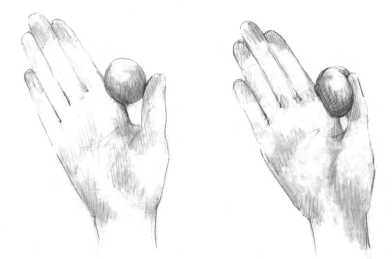

INSTRUCTION: Place putty ball between thumb and index finger of
right hand. Press thumb toward index finger. Repeat
with left hand.

HOLD: _____ second(s) **REPEAT:** _____ time(s) **FREQUENCY:** _____ x/day

SPECIAL PROTOCOLS/NOTES: _____

_____

_____

_____

PATIENT NAME: _____ DATE: _____

THERAPIST NAME: _____

Individual Finger Flexion

PURPOSE: To strengthen front of finger muscles.

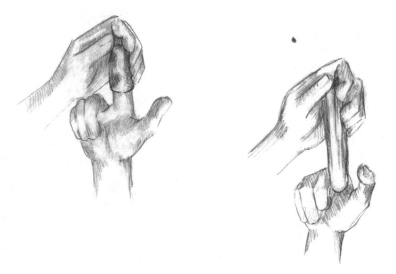

INSTRUCTION: Shape putty into a cylindrical shape and hold with fingers in palm of right hand. Push index finger through the middle of putty. Bend index finger toward body as if signaling someone to come here. Repeat exercise between middle, ring, and pinky finger. Repeat with left hand.

HOLD: _____ second(s) **REPEAT:** _____ time(s) **FREQUENCY:** _____ x/day

SPECIAL PROTOCOLS/NOTES: _____
_____
_____
_____

PATIENT NAME: _____ DATE: _____
THERAPIST NAME: _____

Four Finger Flexion

PURPOSE: To strengthen front of finger muscles.

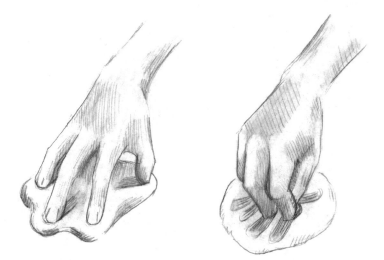

INSTRUCTION: Flatten putty into a pancake. Spread out fingers of right hand and embed fingertips in putty. Pull fingers together. Repeat with left hand.

HOLD: _____ second(s) **REPEAT:** _____ time(s) **FREQUENCY:** _____ x/day

SPECIAL PROTOCOLS/NOTES: _____

_____

_____

_____

PATIENT NAME: _____ DATE: _____

THERAPIST NAME: _____

Individual Finger Extension

PURPOSE: To strengthen back of finger muscles.

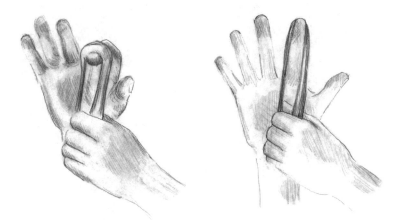

INSTRUCTION: Bend index finger to palm on right hand. Loop putty around index finger. Straighten finger. Repeat with middle, ring, and pinky fingers. Repeat with left hand.

HOLD: _____ second(s)   **REPEAT:** _____ time(s) **FREQUENCY:** _____ x/day

SPECIAL PROTOCOLS/NOTES: _____

_____

_____

_____

PATIENT NAME: _____   DATE: _____

THERAPIST NAME: _____

Four Finger Extension

PURPOSE: To strengthen back of finger muscles.

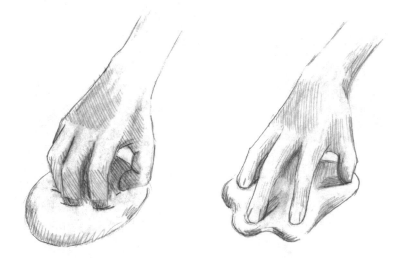

INSTRUCTION: Flatten putty into a pancake. Pull fingers of right hand together and embed tips of fingers in putty. Spread fingers out away from thumb. Repeat with left hand.

HOLD: _____ second(s) **REPEAT:** _____ time(s) **FREQUENCY:** _____ x/day

SPECIAL PROTOCOLS/NOTES: _____

_____

_____

_____

PATIENT NAME: _____ DATE: _____

THERAPIST NAME: _____

Metacarpal Phalangeal Extension

PURPOSE: To strengthen finger muscles.

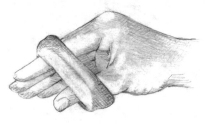
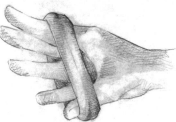

INSTRUCTION: Loop putty around base of fingers and thumb of right hand. Straighten fingers. Squeeze fingers and thumb together. Raise fingers toward ceiling, keeping fingers straight. Repeat with left hand.

HOLD: _____ second(s) **REPEAT:** _____ time(s) **FREQUENCY:** _____ x/day

SPECIAL PROTOCOLS/NOTES: _____

_____

_____

_____

PATIENT NAME: _____ DATE: _____

THERAPIST NAME: _____

Metacarpal Phalangeal Extension and Intrinsic Stretch

PURPOSE: To strengthen muscles at base of fingers and improve range of motion in fingers.

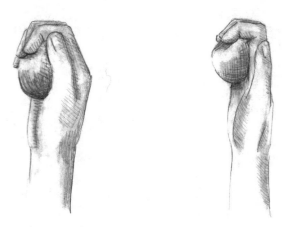

INSTRUCTION: Place putty ball between flexed fingers of right hand. Extend joint at base of fingers. Squeeze fingertips into putty without moving base of fingers. Return to starting position. Repeat with left side.

HOLD: _____ second(s) **REPEAT:** _____ time(s) **FREQUENCY:** _____ x/day

SPECIAL PROTOCOLS/NOTES: _____

_____

_____

_____

PATIENT NAME: _____ DATE: _____

THERAPIST NAME: _____

Finger Abduction

PURPOSE: To strengthen outer finger muscles.

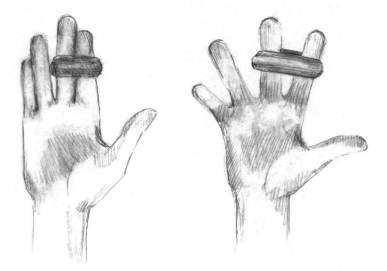

INSTRUCTION: Loop putty around middle of index and middle finger of right hand. Move fingers apart. Repeat exercise with loop around middle of middle finger and ring finger, and ring finger and pinky finger. Repeat with left hand.

HOLD: _____ second(s) **REPEAT:** _____ time(s) **FREQUENCY:** _____ x/day

SPECIAL PROTOCOLS/NOTES: _____

_____

_____

_____

PATIENT NAME: _____ DATE: _____

THERAPIST NAME: _____

Finger Abduction
with Putty Around All Fingers

PURPOSE: To strengthen outer finger muscles.

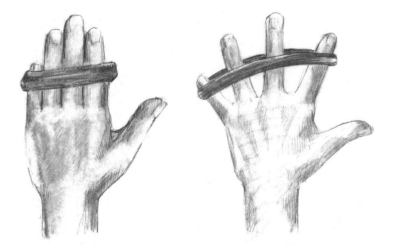

INSTRUCTION: Loop putty around outside of fingers of left hand. Move fingers apart. Repeat with right hand.

HOLD: _____ second(s) **REPEAT:** _____ time(s) **FREQUENCY:** _____ x/day

SPECIAL PROTOCOLS/NOTES: _____

_____

_____

_____

PATIENT NAME: _____ DATE: _____

THERAPIST NAME: _____

Finger Adduction

PURPOSE: To strengthen inner finger muscles.

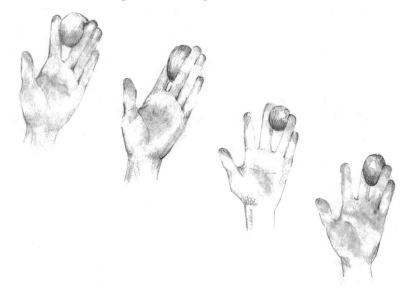

INSTRUCTION: Place putty ball between index and middle finger of right hand. Squeeze ball. Repeat exercise between middle finger and ring finger, and ring finger and pinky finger. Repeat with left hand.

HOLD: _____ second(s) **REPEAT:** _____ time(s) **FREQUENCY:** _____ x/day

SPECIAL PROTOCOLS/NOTES: _____

_____

_____

_____

PATIENT NAME: _____ DATE: _____

THERAPIST NAME: _____

Finger Scissor

PURPOSE: To strengthen finger muscles and increase range of motion and coordination in fingers.

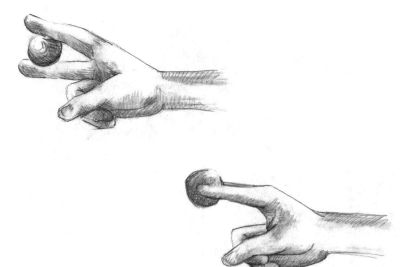

INSTRUCTION: Place ball of putty between index finger and middle finger or right hand. Rotate ball clockwise and counterclockwise. Repeat exercise between middle finger and ring finger, and ring finger and pinky finger. Repeat with left hand.

HOLD: _____ second(s) **REPEAT:** _____ time(s) **FREQUENCY:** _____ x/day

SPECIAL PROTOCOLS/NOTES: _____

_____

_____

_____

PATIENT NAME: _____ DATE: _____

THERAPIST NAME: _____

Wrist Flexion

PURPOSE: To strengthen front side of forearm and wrist muscles.

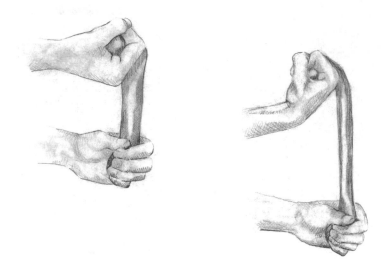

INSTRUCTION: Place right wrist over edge of table with palm up. Place putty in right hand and slip between index and middle finger. Hold other end of putty with left hand. Bend right wrist up toward ceiling. Repeat with left hand.

HOLD: _____ second(s) **REPEAT:** _____ time(s) **FREQUENCY:** _____ x/day

SPECIAL PROTOCOLS/NOTES: Do not lift forearm off table.

_____
_____
_____

PATIENT NAME: _____ DATE: _____

THERAPIST NAME: _____

Wrist Extension

PURPOSE: To strengthen back side of forearm and wrist muscles.

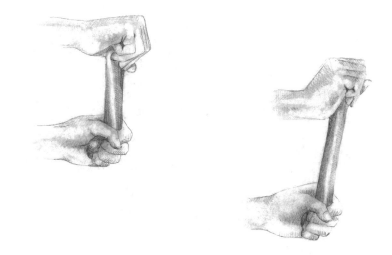

INSTRUCTION: Place right wrist over edge of table with palm down. Grasp one end of putty with right hand and hold other end of putty with left hand. Extend right wrist up toward ceiling. Repeat with left hand.

HOLD: _____ second(s) **REPEAT:** _____ time(s) **FREQUENCY:** _____ x/day

SPECIAL PROTOCOLS/NOTES: Do not lift forearm off table. _____

_____

_____

_____

PATIENT NAME: _____ DATE: _____

THERAPIST NAME: _____

Rolling Pin Roll

PURPOSE: To strengthen finger, forearm, and wrist muscles and improve coordination.

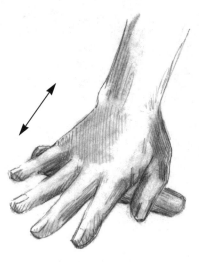

INSTRUCTION: Place a ball of putty on table. With right hand, roll putty back and forth into a cylindrical shape. Repeat with left hand.

HOLD: _____ second(s) **REPEAT:** _____ time(s) **FREQUENCY:** _____ x/day

SPECIAL PROTOCOLS/NOTES: _____
_____
_____
_____

PATIENT NAME: _____ DATE: _____

THERAPIST NAME: _____

Wrist Pronation

PURPOSE: To strengthen forearm and wrist muscles.

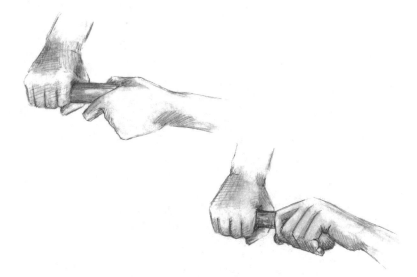

INSTRUCTION: Roll putty into a cylindrical shape. Place both forearms on table. Place putty in left hand, between thumb and index finger, with thumb up. Hold other end of putty with right hand. Rotate wrist counterclockwise, as if unscrewing a light bulb. Repeat with right hand.

HOLD: _____ second(s) **REPEAT:** _____ time(s) **FREQUENCY:** _____ x/day

SPECIAL PROTOCOLS/NOTES: _____

_____

_____

_____

PATIENT NAME: _____ DATE: _____

THERAPIST NAME: _____

Wrist Supination

PURPOSE: To strengthen forearm and wrist muscles.

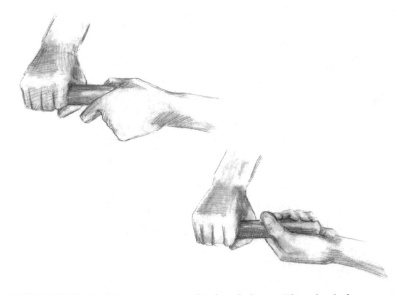

INSTRUCTION: Roll putty into a cylindrical shape. Place both forearms on table. Place putty in left hand with thumb up. Hold other end of putty with right hand. Rotate left wrist clockwise, as if screwing in a light bulb. Repeat with right hand.

HOLD: _____ second(s) **REPEAT:** _____ time(s) **FREQUENCY:** _____ x/day

SPECIAL PROTOCOLS/NOTES: _____

_____

_____

_____

PATIENT NAME: _____ DATE: _____

THERAPIST NAME: _____

Wrist Radial Deviation

PURPOSE: To strengthen forearm and wrist muscles.

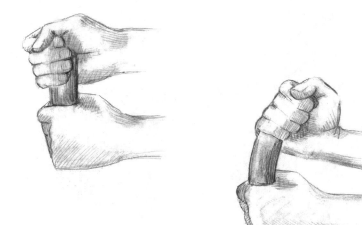

INSTRUCTION: Roll putty into a cylindrical shape. Grasp putty between fingers and palms in both hands with thumbs up and right hand above left hand. Move right hand up away from left hand. Repeat with left hand.

HOLD: _____ second(s) **REPEAT:** _____ time(s) **FREQUENCY:** _____ x/day

SPECIAL PROTOCOLS/NOTES: _____

_____

_____

_____

PATIENT NAME: _____ DATE: _____

THERAPIST NAME: _____

Wrist Ulnar Deviation

PURPOSE: To strengthen forearm and wrist muscles.

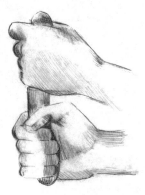

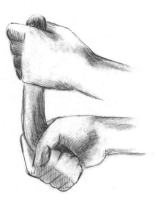

INSTRUCTION: Roll putty into a cylindrical shape. Grasp putty between fingers and palms in both hands with thumbs up and right hand below left hand. Move right hand down from left hand. Repeat with left hand.

HOLD: _____ second(s) **REPEAT:** _____ time(s) **FREQUENCY:** _____ x/day

SPECIAL PROTOCOLS/NOTES: _____
_____
_____
_____

PATIENT NAME: _____ DATE: _____

THERAPIST NAME: _____

RESISTIVE PUTTY EXERCISES

FEET/LOWER EXTREMITY EXERCISES

Metatarsal and Phalangeal Stretch

PURPOSE: To stretch toes and arch of foot.

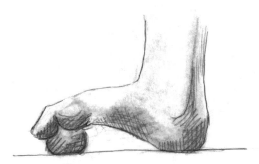

INSTRUCTION: Sit in chair. Place ball of putty on floor under toes of right foot. Curl toes around ball. Repeat with left foot.

HOLD: _____ second(s) **REPEAT:** _____ time(s) **FREQUENCY:** _____ x/day

SPECIAL PROTOCOLS/NOTES: _____

_____

_____

_____

PATIENT NAME: _____ DATE: _____

THERAPIST NAME: _____

Toe Flexion

PURPOSE: To strengthen toe muscles and improve range of motion.

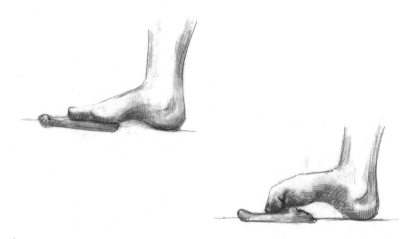

INSTRUCTION: Sit in chair in neutral position. Flatten putty ball into a pancake and place on floor. Place right forefoot on putty pancake. Curl toes toward heel. Repeat with left foot.

HOLD: _____ second(s) **REPEAT:** _____ time(s) **FREQUENCY:** _____ x/day

SPECIAL PROTOCOLS/NOTES: Do not lift foot off floor.
_____
_____
_____
_____

PATIENT NAME: _____ DATE: _____
THERAPIST NAME: _____

Toe Extension

PURPOSE: To strengthen toe muscles and improve range of motion.

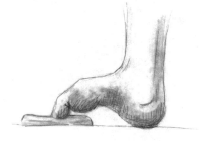
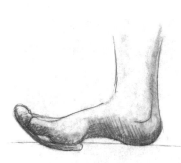

INSTRUCTION: Sit in chair in neutral position. Flatten putty ball into a pancake and place on floor. Curl toes of right foot toward heel and place on putty pancake. Straighten and bend toes up toward knee. Keep forefoot on putty. Repeat with left foot.

HOLD: _____ second(s) **REPEAT:** _____ time(s) **FREQUENCY:** _____ x/day

SPECIAL PROTOCOLS/NOTES: Do not lift foot off floor. _____
_____
_____
_____

PATIENT NAME: _____ DATE: _____

THERAPIST NAME: _____

Toe Flick with Putty Ball

PURPOSE: To strengthen toe muscles and increase range of motion.

INSTRUCTION: Sit in chair. Curl toes of right foot under. Place ball of putty in front of toes. Flick ball with toes. Repeat with left foot.

HOLD: _____ second(s) **REPEAT:** _____ time(s) **FREQUENCY:** _____ x/day

SPECIAL PROTOCOLS/NOTES: _____

_____

_____

_____

PATIENT NAME: _____ DATE: _____

THERAPIST NAME: _____

Toe Adduction

PURPOSE: To strengthen inner toe muscles.

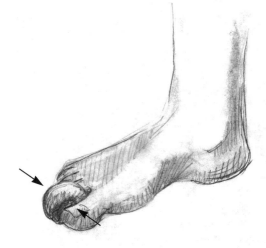

INSTRUCTION: Sit in chair in neutral position. Place small putty ball between great toe and second toe of right foot. Squeeze putty ball. Repeat exercise placing putty ball between second and third toes, and between fourth and fifth toes. Repeat with left foot.

HOLD: _____ second(s) **REPEAT:** _____ time(s) **FREQUENCY:** _____ x/day

SPECIAL PROTOCOLS/NOTES: _____
_____
_____
_____

PATIENT NAME: _____ DATE: _____

THERAPIST NAME: _____

Knee Flexion/Extension with Putty Ball

PURPOSE: To strengthen ankle and leg muscles and improve coordination.

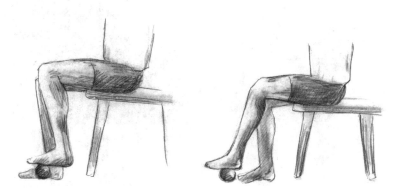

INSTRUCTION: Sit on chair. Place putty ball under toes of left foot. Straighten left knee until ball rolls to heel. Roll ball back and forth between toes and heel in a rapid, rhythmic pattern. Repeat with right foot.

HOLD: _____ second(s) **REPEAT:** _____ time(s) **FREQUENCY:** _____ x/day

SPECIAL PROTOCOLS/NOTES: Rest foot lightly on putty ball. Try not to flatten putty ball.

_____

PATIENT NAME: _____ DATE: _____

THERAPIST NAME: _____

Hip Internal/External Rotation

PURPOSE: To strengthen ankle, hip, and leg muscles and improve range of motion.

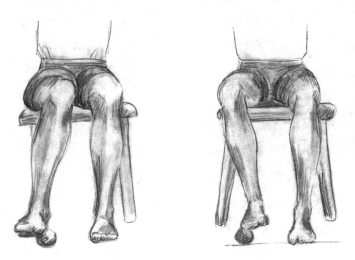

INSTRUCTION: Sit on chair in neutral position. Place putty ball under right forefoot. Roll ball to inside and outside of foot in a rapid, rhythmic pattern. Repeat with left foot.

HOLD: _____ second(s) **REPEAT:** _____ time(s) **FREQUENCY:** _____ x/day

SPECIAL PROTOCOLS/NOTES: Rest foot lightly on putty ball. Try not to flatten putty ball.

_____

_____

PATIENT NAME: _____ DATE: _____

THERAPIST NAME: _____

CHAPTER ELEVEN

Case
Studies

CASE STUDY ONE

WRITTEN BY: Barbara J. Headley, M.S., P.T.
sEMG Instructor and owner of Movement
Assessment, Research and Education Center,
Boulder, CO

Exercise is the foundation upon which physical therapy and rehabilitation in general is built. The use of various resistive devices for strengthening has been a part of rehabilitation since the first strengthening exercise was prescribed. The foundation of exercise programs has been the biomechanical assessment of a muscle's origin, insertion, structural design, and relationship to the joint or joints that it crosses. From this framework, physics provides us with information about how much force a muscle might be able to generate during a given movement pattern, and which muscles are better designed for tasks within a certain range of motion. From this, a list of prime movers and assistant movers has been compiled for a given movement pattern. Therapists then select and design exercise programs to fit such needs as: 1) strengthening for power, 2) endurance training, 3) strengthening for static work or, 4) strengthening for eccentric tasks.

The addition of resistance to an exercise is a critical element in strengthening a muscle. The assumption has been that if the movement can be accomplished when resistance is added, then the prime movers have responded appropriately to the loading and strengthening is occurring. This assumption, however, is not always true. The use of surface electromyography (sEMG) allows us to examine many muscles during movement. There is often a vast difference between how a healthy, asymptomatic subject responds to the resistive task as compared to how a patient responds. The element of greatest variation is that of motor control strategies. Pain from an injury can change soft tissue length, tone, and the ability to respond properly to loading. Muscles that are the expected prime movers of a particular task may be totally inhibited, or may respond appropriately to active exercise, only to succumb to protective inhibition when the task is resisted. The inhibition may be local, i.e., an active trigger point, or it may be the result of central drive changes. In the latter case, the motor control strategy is altered due to the pain and adaptive movement strategies developed, often to give the injured tissue time to heal. These adaptive motor plans may persist and the patient can develop pain from these altered patterns, the original injury long since healed.

Exercise is dependent, therefore, upon thorough examination of how the patient is responding to the challenge of resistive exercise. An improper response may lead to additional pain and even new injury to tissues that adapt to perform the task but are poorly designed to do so for long periods of time.

In the first exercise for which sEMG data is provided—shoulder flexion—the anterior deltoid is a vital component to this exercise being done with proper biomechanical forces on the joint. The amplitude of the anterior deltoid is almost double the amplitude of the same movement without resistance. Many of the patients I see perform shoulder flexion exhibit almost total inhibition of this muscle, altering the forces on the joint and requiring significant changes in the activation of surrounding muscles. As therapists, it is our decision whether or not a patient should be given an exercise with such adaptive changes.

Exercise may be used to correct postural dysfunction, increase the efficiency of a particular movement pattern, or assist in rebalancing shortened and lengthened muscles. Exercises may be designed to achieve greater relaxation of muscles following their contraction or to strengthen a particular muscle or group of muscles. The use of sEMG can be critical in determining whether or not the muscle to be strengthened is responding in the appropriate fashion. Fatigue analysis with sEMG can assist in establishing when the muscle has recovered after an exercise session, guiding the therapist to completion of treatment goals with minimal setbacks due to inhibition, delayed onset muscle soreness, failure to recover, or even new injury.

Synopsis of microvolt readings for five resistive band exercises

	Pectoralis Major	Anterior Deltoid	Posterior Deltoid	Serratus Anterior	Upper Trapezius	Supra-Spinatus	Infra-Spinatus	Lower Trapezius
Standing Unilateral Shoulder Flexion	858	1288	669	1031	2883	1913	648	1617
Standing Shoulder Abduction to 90°	92	428	436	600	2265	2150	532	1110
Standing Shoulder Abduction to 180°	1849	1893	943	1376	3200	2058	887	1027
Standing Shoulder PNF D2 – Extension	237	409	1531	285	524	1019	406	564
Sitting Shoulder PNF D2 – Flexion on Ball	589	1073	1132	1087	555	1039	1185	1106

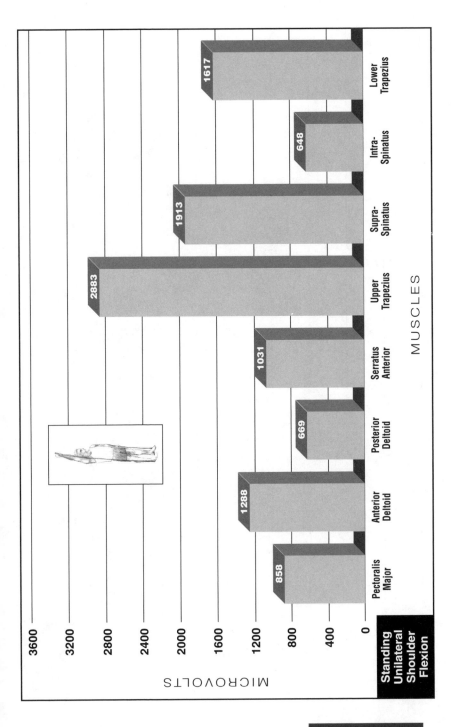

Standing Unilateral Shoulder Flexion

MUSCLES

MICROVOLTS

Muscle	Value
Pectoralis Major	858
Anterior Deltoid	1288
Posterior Deltoid	669
Serratus Anterior	1031
Upper Trapezius	2883
Supra-Spinatus	1913
Intra-Spinatus	648
Lower Trapezius	1617

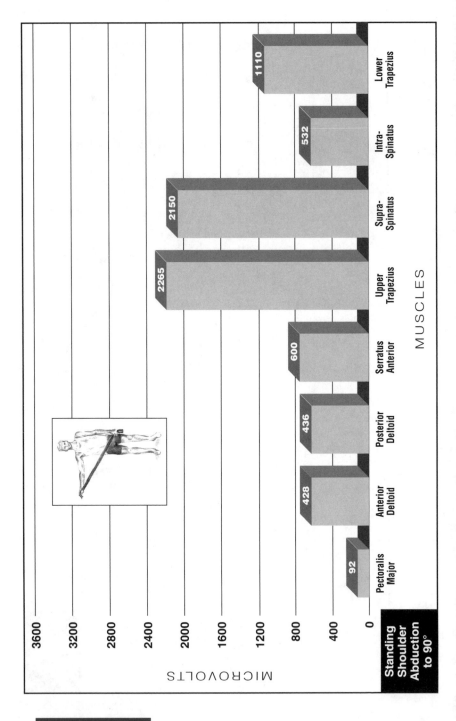

MICROVOLTS

| | 3600 | 3200 | 2800 | 2400 | 2000 | 1600 | 1200 | 800 | 400 | 0 |

Standing Shoulder Abduction to 90°

MUSCLES

- Pectoralis Major: 92
- Anterior Deltoid: 428
- Posterior Deltoid: 436
- Serratus Anterior: 600
- Upper Trapezius: 2265
- Supra-Spinatus: 2150
- Intra-Spinatus: 532
- Lower Trapezius: 1110

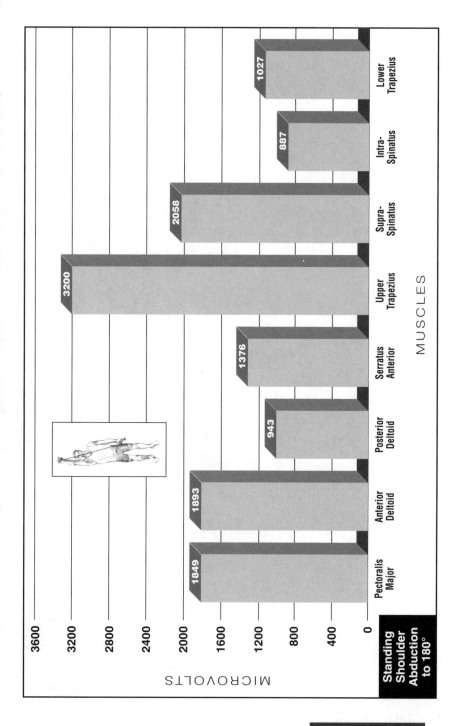

Standing Shoulder Abduction to 180°

MICROVOLTS

MUSCLES

Pectoralis Major: 1849
Anterior Deltoid: 1893
Posterior Deltoid: 943
Serratus Anterior: 1376
Upper Trapezius: 3200
Supra-Spinatus: 2058
Intra-Spinatus: 887
Lower Trapezius: 1027

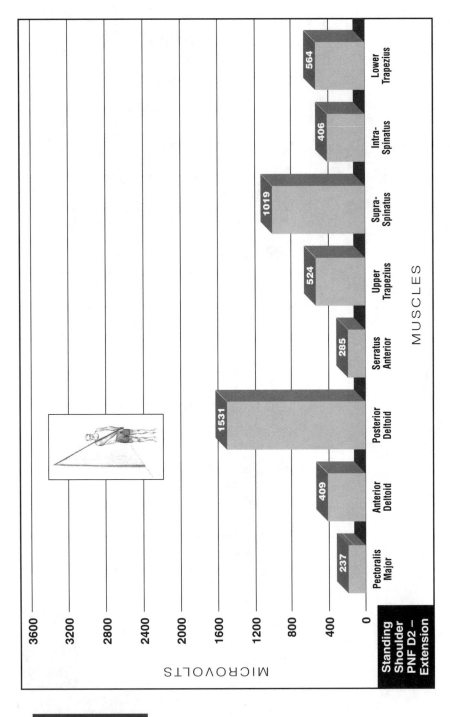

MICROVOLTS

3600
3200
2800
2400
2000
1600
1200
800
400
0

| Standing Shoulder PNF D2 – Extension |

Pectoralis Major — 237
Anterior Deltoid — 409
Posterior Deltoid — 1531
Serratus Anterior — 285
Upper Trapezius — 524
Supra-Spinatus — 1019
Intra-Spinatus — 406
Lower Trapezius — 564

MUSCLES

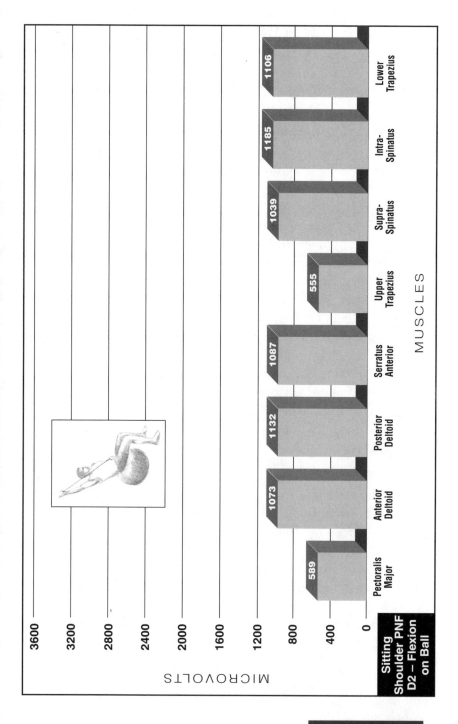

Sitting Shoulder PNF D2 – Flexion on Ball

MICROVOLTS

MUSCLES

Muscle	Microvolts
Pectoralis Major	589
Anterior Deltoid	1073
Posterior Deltoid	1132
Serratus Anterior	1087
Upper Trapezius	555
Supra-Spinatus	1039
Intra-Spinatus	1185
Lower Trapezius	1106

CASE STUDY TWO

WRITTEN BY: Leslie Vail, P.T.
Owner of Colorado Physical Therapy,
Greeley, CO

DIAGNOSIS: Bilateral Shoulder Impingement

HISTORY

Thirty-three-year-old male reports to physical therapy clinic complaining of bilateral shoulder pain. He states he had a shoulder decompression and bursa removal in the right shoulder in January 1983. Patient reports shoulder pain began about one year ago while practicing a lot of golf. He describes his pain as being "on top of the right shoulder" (in the area of the acromioclavicular joint) with sharp pain in the posterior shoulder with activities. The left shoulder presents the same symptoms, but he complains of referred pain to the left ring finger. The left shoulder bothers him more than the right when golfing. Patient states his goal is to be pain free while playing golf.

EVALUATION

OBJECTIVE FINDINGS: Active Range of Motion (AROM): cervical spine Within Normal Limits (WNL); right and left shoulder internal rotation (IR) 0–65 degrees, external rotation (ER) WNL, abduction 0–160, flexion 0–160; Noted that patient was unable to extend his left elbow fully with full AROM of the shoulder, however his AROM was WNL when tested separately. Strength: left and right tricep 4/5, bicep 4/5, shoulder abduction at 90 degrees 4-/5, serratus anterior 4/5, supraspinatus 4-/5, ER 4-/5, lower trapezius 3+/5; left IR 3+/5, and rhomboid 4/5; right IR 4-/5, and rhomboid 5/5.

POSTURE: Patient was noted to have a flattened thoracic spine curve without a scoliosis. He stands with arms forward and internally rotated. The left scapula was abducted 1 cm further from midline than the right scapula. Hypertrophy in right rhomboid and atrophy in left lower trapezius muscle noted. Flexibility length of the latisimus dorsi was 120 degrees of shoulder flexion measured in supine with lower back extension locked out. Patient was also noted to stand with an anterior pelvic tilt and forward head.

PALPATION: No cervical or upper thoracic mechanical dysfunctions were noted. The left clavicle was posteriorly rotated with arms in neutral position. The left SC joint depressed beyond normal with shoulder shrugs. Palpation to the shoulder tissues revealed tenderness in the supraspinatus, infraspinatus, and subscapularus muscles. Patient was tender over the anterior shoulder tissues with a forward humerus noted bilaterally.

SPECIAL TESTS: Positive impingement test bilaterally, positive relocation test bilaterally, negative Adson's test, negative grind test, negative drop arm test, negative Long's test.

TREATMENT ONE

Patient received education and corrective exercises for posture and scapular stabilization recruitment. Patient was issued a 3-inch-diameter foam roller and instructed in a home exercise program which included pectoralis stretches and scapular down and ins for lower trapezius recruitment. McConnell taping techniques were then used for glenohumeral relocation to help facilitate the humerus into a neutral position during scapular re-ed exercises.

At the end of the first treatment, patient was noted to have improved posture in standing with his arms hanging in neutral position at his sides.

TREATMENT TWO

Patient was able to successfully recruit his lower trapezius muscle. He was also able to maintain neutral posture with verbal cueing, however with difficulty secondary to shoulder weakness and tightness. Patient received muscle energy techniques, myofascial release techniques, and ball exercises.

At the end of treatment, patient had active shoulder range of motion with decreased impingement pain. He continues to have a scapular posture problem.

TREATMENT THREE

Patient reports increased shoulder mobility and he states his shoulder is feeling the best it has since his surgery in 1983. His left shoulder continues to bother him with continued pain in the anterior shoulder. The left shoulder presented in an abducted and tilted position at rest, however was corrected to neutral with verbal cueing. Patient received ultrasound (US), soft tissue mobilization (STM), myofascial release (MFR) techniques, and McConnell taping to shoulders bilaterally. His home exercise program was not progressed.

TREATMENT FOUR

Patient reported continued resolution of right shoulder pain and now has decreased left shoulder pain. The tenderness in the left anterior shoulder is lessening to palpation. Patient received US, STM, and MFR. Patient was instructed in abdominal stabilization and red Theraband® exercises for his home program: wall push-ups, shoulder internal/external stretches (5 stretches daily), and bilateral external rotation in neutral (3 sets of 10 repetitions daily).

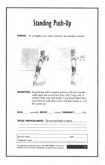

TREATMENT FIVE

Patient reported no left shoulder pain secondary to impingement. He strained his right shoulder while doing household chores, however felt better during this treatment. A quick assessment of the shoulder reveals improved scapular position, and decreased pectoralis and latisimus tightness. Weakness in the serratus anterior and shoulder stabilizers continued and ball exercises were started.

TREATMENT SIX

Improvements noted in posture, and strength in the serratus anterior, lower trapezius, and internal and external rotators. The left humerous is still noted to be minimally forward. The patient was instructed in the following red Thera-Band® exercises: supraspinatus exercise (30 repetitions), shoulder internal and external rotations at 90 degrees abduction (10–15 repetitions each).

TREATMENT SEVEN

Patient reported that his shoulders feel the best they have since he can remember. He is anxious to start golfing again, but was advised to refer to the outline of recommended golfing activities he could begin in two weeks. He was instructed in the following resistive band exercises: golf swing (15 repetitions), elbow flexion and elbow extension (15 repetitions), and sitting bilateral shoulder rowing in trunk flexion (15 repetitions).

Patient was issued green and blue Thera-Band® to use as he gains strength in his shoulders. He was instructed to increase to 3 sets of 15 before moving to the next color of resistance.

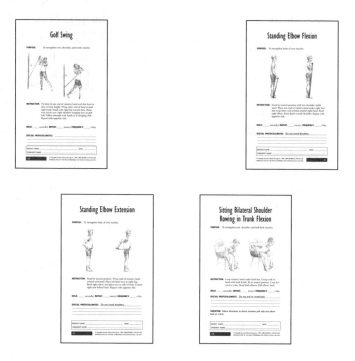

OUTCOME

Patient did not receive any further therapy for his shoulders, because he moved out of state. He did, however, stop by the clinic and report that he was able to play 18 holes of golf, pain free. He stated that he continues to do his exercises 3 times a week for maintenance.

CASE STUDY THREE

WRITTEN BY: Caroline Corning Creager, P.T.
Swiss Ball, Resistive Band, Foam Roller, and
B.O.I.N.G. Instructor, Owner of Executive
Physical Therapy, Inc., Berthoud, CO.

DIAGNOSIS: Left distal radial fracture into growth plate
and joint

HISTORY

The author sustained a left radial fracture after falling on a hyperextended wrist while playing soccer. (She has had no history of previous injuries to her wrist, elbow, or shoulder). Her left arm was casted above the elbow, in elbow and slight wrist flexion for three weeks; followed by a below elbow cast, in neutral position, for three weeks. She experienced minimal to moderate swelling in arm, forearm, and hand during the six weeks she wore a cast.

EVALUATION

Minimal swelling noted in left anterior and posterior distal radial region, and minimal discomfort in same region with palpation was reported. Strength was not tested secondary to pain.

The following active range of motion measurements were taken two and twelve weeks following the removal of her second cast:

ACTIVE RANGE OF MOTION MEASUREMENTS

	Two weeks s/p cast removal		Twelve weeks s/p cast removal	
	Left	Right	Left	Right
Wrist Flexion	43	90	84	91
Wrist Extension	35 pain*	62	58	62
Pronation	86	90	90	90
Supination	80 pain*	90	88	90

*pain noted in the left distal radial region

Grip strength measurements were taken with a hand-held dynamometer, and by manual muscle tests, five weeks' and twelve weeks' status post removal of her second cast:

	Five weeks s/p cast removal		Twelve weeks s/p cast removal	

HAND-HELD DYNAMOMETER
GRIP STRENGTH MEASUREMENTS

	Left	Right	Left	Right
Setting #1	22# pain*	56#	49#	60#
Setting #2	34# discomfort*	75#	50#	70#
Setting #3	28# pain*	84#	55#	81#
Setting #4	35# discomfort*	78#	68#	83#
Setting #5	31# discomfort*	62#	55#	63#
Average of all five settings	30#	71#	53#	73#

MANUAL MUSCLE TEST
STRENGTH MEASUREMENTS

	Left	Right	Left	Right
Wrist Flexion	3+/5 pain*	5/5	4+/5	5/5
Wrist Extension	3+/5 pain*	"	4+/5	"
Pronation	3+/5	"	4+/5	"
Supination	3-/5	"	4/5	"
Elbow Flexion	4-/5	"	4+/5	"
Elbow Extension	4+/5	"	5-/5	"

TREATMENT

The author was on a self-directed independent exercise and treatment program. She performed massage for swelling reduction and friction massage to break down scar tissue. Ice was applied as necessary for swelling reduction. She exercised three to five days a week, from 10 minutes to 20 minutes a day using resistive bands, resistive putty, Swiss balls, foam rollers and the B.O.I.N.G. She used many of the exercises in this book, however, the following exercises were used consistently throughout her exercise regimen.

Sitting Wrist Flexion

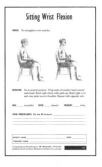

INSTRUCTION: Sit in neutral position. Wrap ends of resistive band around each hand. Bend right elbow with palm up. Bend right wrist and raise palm toward shoulder. Repeat with opposite side.

HOLD: ____ second(s)   REPEAT: ____ time(s)   FREQUENT: ____ x/day

SPECIAL PRECAUTIONS/NOTES: Do not lift forearm. ____

PATIENT NAME: ____   DATE: ____
THERAPIST NAME: ____

Sitting Wrist Extension

PURPOSE: To strengthen wrist muscles.

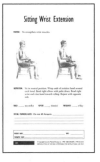

INSTRUCTION: Sit in neutral position. Wrap ends of resistive band around each hand. Bend right elbow with palm down. Bend right wrist and raise hand toward ceiling. Repeat with opposite side.

HOLD: ____ second(s)   REPEAT: ____ time(s)   FREQUENT: ____ x/day

SPECIAL PRECAUTIONS/NOTES: Do not lift forearm. ____

PATIENT NAME: ____   DATE: ____
THERAPIST NAME: ____

Sitting Wrist Radial Deviation in Neutral

PURPOSE: To strengthen wrist muscles.

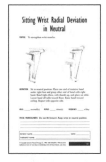

INSTRUCTION: Sit in neutral position. Place one end of resistive band under right foot and grasp other end of band with right hand. Bend right elbow, with thumb up, and place on table. Lower hand off table toward floor. Raise hand toward ceiling. Repeat with opposite side.

HOLD: ____ second(s)   REPEAT: ____ time(s)   FREQUENT: ____ x/day

SPECIAL PRECAUTIONS/NOTES: Do not lift forearm. Keep wrist in neutral position. ____

PATIENT NAME: ____   DATE: ____
THERAPIST NAME: ____

Sitting Wrist Ulnar Deviation in Neutral

PURPOSE: To strengthen wrist muscles.

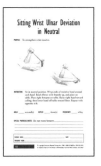

INSTRUCTION: Sit in neutral position. Wrap ends of resistive band around each hand. Bend elbows with thumbs up, and place on table. Place right forearm on table. Raise right hand toward ceiling, then lower hand off table toward floor. Repeat with opposite side.

HOLD: ____ second(s)   REPEAT: ____ time(s)   FREQUENT: ____ x/day

SPECIAL PRECAUTIONS/NOTES: Do not move forearm. ____

PATIENT NAME: ____   DATE: ____
THERAPIST NAME: ____

Wrist Pronation

PURPOSE: To strengthen forearm and wrist muscles.

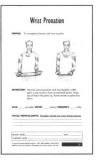

INSTRUCTION: Stand in neutral position with feet shoulder-width apart. Loop resistive band around both hands. Grasp top of loop with palms up. Rotate hands so palms face down.

HOLD: ____ second(s)   REPEAT: ____ time(s)   FREQUENCY: ____ x/day

SPECIAL PROTOCOLS/NOTES: Shoulders should not move during exercise.

PATIENT NAME: ____   DATE: ____
THERAPIST NAME: ____

Wrist Supination

PURPOSE: To strengthen forearm and wrist muscles.

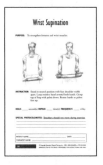

INSTRUCTION: Stand in neutral position with feet shoulder-width apart. Loop resistive band around both hands. Grasp top of loop with palms down. Rotate hands so palms face up.

HOLD: ____ second(s)   REPEAT: ____ time(s)   FREQUENCY: ____ x/day

SPECIAL PROTOCOLS/NOTES: Shoulders should not move during exercise.

PATIENT NAME: ____   DATE: ____
THERAPIST NAME: ____

Standing Shoulder External Rotation

PURPOSE: To strengthen shoulder muscles.

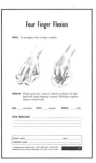

INSTRUCTION: Tie knot in one end of resistive band and shut knot in door or close to it. Stand in neutral position with right side facing knot. Wrap other end of band around left hand. Bend left elbow and move hand away from abdomen. Repeat with opposite side.

HOLD: ____ second(s)   REPEAT: ____ time(s)   FREQUENCY: ____ x/day

SPECIAL PROTOCOLS/NOTES: Do not slouch.

PATIENT NAME: ____   DATE: ____
THERAPIST NAME: ____

Prone Shoulder Rowing on Ball

PURPOSE: To strengthen mid-back and shoulder muscles.

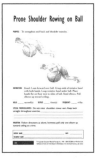

INSTRUCTION: Kneel. Lean forward over ball. Grasp ends of resistive band with both hands. Loop resistive band under ball. Place hands flat on floor next to sides of ball. Stand elbows. Pull elbows up toward ceiling.

HOLD: ____ second(s)   REPEAT: ____ time(s)   FREQUENCY: ____ x/day

SPECIAL PROTOCOLS/NOTES: Do not raise shoulders above ears. Keep back straight throughout exercise.

VARIATION: Follow directions as above, however, pull only one elbow up toward ceiling at a time.

PATIENT NAME: ____   DATE: ____
THERAPIST NAME: ____

Prone Push-Up

PURPOSE: To strengthen arm, forearm, and shoulder muscles.

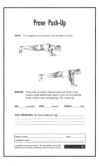

INSTRUCTION: Wrap ends of resistive band around each hand. Loop resistive band behind back. Kneel. Lean forward placing hands on floor and extending legs. Do a push-up.

HOLD: ____ second(s)   REPEAT: ____ time(s)   FREQUENCY: ____ x/day

SPECIAL PROTOCOLS/NOTES: Do not abdomen sag.

PATIENT NAME: ____   DATE: ____
THERAPIST NAME: ____

Four Finger Flexion

PURPOSE: To strengthen flexor of finger muscles.

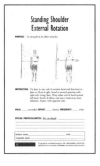

INSTRUCTION: Flatten putty into a pancake. Spread out fingers of right hand and embed fingertips in putty. Pull fingers together. Repeat with left hand.

HOLD: ____ second(s)   REPEAT: ____ time(s)   FREQUENT: ____ x/day

SPECIAL PRECAUTIONS: ____

PATIENT NAME: ____   DATE: ____
THERAPIST NAME: ____

Four Finger Extension

PURPOSE: To strengthen back of finger muscles.

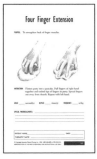

INSTRUCTION: Flatten putty into a pancake. Pull fingers of right hand together and embed tips of fingers in putty. Spread fingers out away from thumb. Repeat with left hand.

HOLD: ____ second(s)   REPEAT: ____ time(s)   FREQUENT: ____ x/day

SPECIAL PRECAUTIONS: ____

PATIENT NAME: ____   DATE: ____
THERAPIST NAME: ____

Putty Ball Squeeze with Hand

PURPOSE: To strengthen flexor muscles in hand.

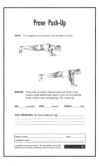

INSTRUCTION: Place putty ball in right hand. Squeeze ball with fingers and thumb. Repeat with left hand.

HOLD: ____ second(s)   REPEAT: ____ time(s)   FREQUENCY: ____ x/day

SPECIAL PROTOCOLS/NOTES: ____

PATIENT NAME: ____   DATE: ____
THERAPIST NAME: ____

OUTCOME:

Twelve weeks' status post cast removal, the author, had no complaints of pain with active range of motion or with any weight-bearing positions. She did report intermittent "catching" of scar tissue with supination of left wrist. Her left wrist active range-of-motion measurements increased 5 to 95 percent, her average left grip strength measurements with the hand-held dynamometer improved by 87 percent, and her left upper extremity manual muscle test measurements increased by at least one full grade for all muscles tested.

References

"Are You Allergic to Latex?" *Safety+Health*, May 1998, p. 63.

Atkinson, Hilary and Deane, Andree. *The Dyna-band Challenge; A Fabulous Figure in Only 10 Minutes a Day.* Woodstock, NY: The Overlook Press, 1991.

Creager, Caroline. *Therapeutic Exercises Using Foam Rollers.* Berthoud, CO: Executive Physical Therapy, Inc., 1996.

Creager, Caroline. *Therapeutic Exercises Using the Swiss Ball.* Berthoud, CO: Executive Physical Therapy, Inc., 1994.

Hintermeister, Robert and Bey, Michael, et al. "Quantification of Elastic Resistance Knee Rehabilitation Exercises." *JOSPT* 28(1): 1988, 40–50.

Houston, Sandy, and Campagna, Phil. *Tubing: A New Way to a Great Shape!* Dartmouth, NH: Fitness Communication, 1985.

Hulme, Janet. *Beyond Kegels: Fabulous four exercises and more to prevent and treat incontinence.* Missoula, MT: Phoenix Publishing Co., 1997.

The Hygenic Corporation. *Thera-Band System of Progressive Resistance, Instruction Manual*, 3rd Edition. Akron, OH: The Hygenic Corporation, 1996.

Kedjidjian, Catherine. "Get the Facts About Latex." *Safety+Health*, May 1998, pp. 58–62.

Lockard, Joanne. "Living with a Latex Allergy." *PT Magazine*, March 1998, pp. 36–42.

Maitland, G.D. *Vertebral Manipulation*, 5th Edition. Butterworth & Co. Ltd., 1986.

Mikesky, Alan and Topp, Robert, et al. "Efficacy of a Home-Based Training Program for Older Adults Using Elastic Tubing." *E J Appl Physiol Occup Physiol.* 69: 1994, pp. 316–320.

Mostardi, Richard and Chapman, Elizabeth. "Improvement in Muscular Strength with the Use of Wide Width Therapeutic Resistive Bands." Akron, OH: Akron City Hospital and The University of Akron.

Page, Philip and Lamberth, John, et al. "Posterior Rotator Cuff Strengthening Using Thera-Band in a Functional Diagonal Pattern in Collegiate Baseball Pitchers." *Athletic Training, NATA* 28(4): 1993, pp. 346–354.

Topp, Robert and Mikesky, Alan, et. al. " The Effect of a 12-Week Dynamic Resistance Strength Training Program on Gait Velocity and Balance of Older Adults." *Gerontol.* 33(4): 1993, pp. 501–506.

Webb, Tamilee. *Tamilee Webb's Original Rubber Band Workout.* New York, NY: Workman Publishing Company, Inc., 1986.

Wynn, Kimberly E. "Going Latex Safe." *PT Magazine*, March 1998, pp. 44, 46–49.

Recommended Reading

 Creager, Caroline Corning. *Bounce Back Into Shape After Baby*, Berthoud, CO: Executive Physical Therapy Inc., 2001.

 Creager, Caroline Corning. *The Airobic Ball™ Strengthening Workout*, Berthoud, CO: Executive Physical Therapy Inc., 1994.

 Creager, Caroline Corning. *The Airobic Ball™ Stretching Workout*, Berthoud, CO: Executive Physical Therapy Inc., 1995.

 Creager, Caroline Corning. *Therapeutic Exercises Using Foam Rollers*, Berthoud, CO: Executive Physical Therapy Inc., 1996.

 Creager, Caroline Corning. *Therapeutic Exercises Using the Swiss Ball*, Berthoud, CO: Executive Physical Therapy Inc., 1994.

Ordering Information

To obtain more information about ordering exercise balls and books please call the following distributors:

AUSTRALIA
Healthtrek: 0500 888843, www.healthtrek.net   OR
Star Systems: 02 6772 7433, www.starsystems.com.au

NEW ZEALAND
Network for Fitness Professionals: 09 479 8635
Email: info@netfitpro.co.nz

SOUTH AFRICA
Thera Med: 27 11 8046746, home.global.co.za/~dhtgo/

UNITED KINGDOM
Russell Medical: 01684 311 444
Email: enquiries@russellmedical.co.uk   OR
Physical Company Ltd: 01494 769 222
www.physicalcompany.co.uk

UNITED STATES & CANADA
Orthopedic Physical Therapy Products:
(800) 367-7393 or (763) 553-0452, www.optp.com

Visit our website at:
www.CarolineCreager.com

Hosting an
Open & Closed Chain
Stabilization Course,
Swiss Ball,
and/or
Foam Roller Courses

by Caroline Corning Creager, P.T.

If you are interested in hosting an open and closed chain course, Swiss ball, or foam roller course, please call 1-800-530-6878 or 970-532-2533, or write to Executive Physical Therapy, Inc., at the address listed below:

Executive Physical Therapy, Inc.
P.O. Box 1319
Berthoud, CO 80513

or e-mail Caroline Corning Creager at:

Caroline_Creager@unforgettable.com

Visit our web site at:

www.CarolineCreager.com

Index

coordination, 19, 249
coughing, 21
Creager, Caroline Corning, iii
crunch, 231
curl, 232

D
deltoids, 31; *see also* shoulder
  muscles and back muscles
demyelinating disease, 19
distal radial fracture, 354
dizziness, 8, 9

E
eczema, 9, 21
elbows, 51-55, 125-127, 245

F
finger muscles, 287-293, 301-
  305, 316-325, 328
fly, 78
foot muscles, 271, 272, 333-340
forearm muscles, 34, 35, 53, 79,
  184, 185, 262, 268, 270, 276,
  277, 297, 298, 326, 327, 329-
  332
free throw, 262

G
gastrocnemius, 41, 42
gluteus medius, 16
golf swing, 266

H
hamstrings, 16, 41
hand muscles, 34, 282-332
hay fever symptoms, 9, 21
hemiplegia, 18
hip muscles, 98, 99, 101-107,

151, 152, 154, 155, 157, 158,
  189, 190, 199-204, 233-244,
  248, 249, 267, 340
hooklying position, 237
hosting a course, 361

I
iliotibial band, 16, 38
indications, 8
inflammation, 10, 11, 14, 15
itching, 9, 21

K
Kegel exercises, 156, 204, 242
kick boxing, 267
knees, 109-113, 159-161, 173,
  191-193, 238, 252, 339
knot-tying techniques, 7

L
lateral epicondylitis, 11
latex allergies, 21-22
latex-free resistive bands, 21
latisimus dorsi, 61, 62
lawnmower pull, 85
leg muscles, 93-99, 101-104,
  165, 166, 168,179, 180, 245-
  249, 251, 252, 263, 267, 271-
  275, 280, 339, 340
Leukopore tape, 21
levator scapulae, 30
lightheadedness, 8
low back pain, 14

M
McConnell tape, 21
microvolt readings, 344-349
mid-scapular, 183
motor loss, 18